Brain Health and the Arts:

ART SMART

A Look at the Brain, Learning, the Arts, and Mental Agility

Lauretta DeForge

DeForge Communications
Portland, Oregon

Copyright © 2004 by Lauretta DeForge

All rights reserved. This publication may not be reproduced by any process without the prior written consent of the author.

Library of Congress Control Number
2004096188

ISBN Number 0-9677846-9-7

Special Acknowledgment

Special thanks to these people for reading my manuscript and giving me feedback: Mark DeForge, Shirley Humphreys, Paul Kerley, Andria Lishka, Jessica Morrell, and Colleen Yechout.

DeForge Communications
http://home.
netcom.com
/ldeforge/

Maunfactured in the United States

First Edition

Introduction

With all the new technology available today to study the brain, one thing has become absolutely clear: How we use our brains determines what kind of brains we have. If we do not lay down the foundations for skills at the correct times, we cannot build on them later. We must continually feed our brains quality stimuli, new stimuli, from our births to our deaths, because it is this stream of mental data which keeps our brains functioning normally.

The search for stimulation is a long-term process. It cannot be avoided or disregarded. As we live longer, we have ever greater opportunities to keep our minds active and useful. We have continually more possibilities for learning, creativity, and development in the arts.

It is my belief that the search for mental stimulation to keep our brains in shape drives humanity. It leads us into creativity and the arts which will be a focus of this book. I give a brief explanation of the brain, our senses, our need for stimulation, creativity, learning, and the arts. It is all of these elements which make our lives richer and keep the brain in top form.

Please check out the bibliography in the back of the book; there are many books you will want to read.

Chapter One 4

Table of Contents

Introduction		p. 3
Chapter 1	Brain Evolution	p. 6
Chapter 2	The Senses	p. 19
Chapter 3	Processing Stimuli	p. 34
Chapter 4	Mental Stimulation, Learning, and the child	p. 61
Chapter 5	Creativity	p. 89
Chapter 6	The Arts and the Four Stages of Life	p. 97
Chapter 7	Mental Stimulation and the Arts	p. 105
Chapter 8	Music and Other Arts	p. 127
Chapter 9	Mental Stimulation and Quality of Life	p. 166
Epilogue	Working to Keep the Brain in Balance	p. 174

Chapter One 5

Appendix I	Future Developments	p. 201
Appendix II	Brain Image Technology	p. 214
Notes	The Author	p. 217
Bibliography		p. 219
Index		p. 228
Order Blank		p. 232

Chapter I

BRAIN EVOLUTION

The power of the human brain is phenomenal. A fruit fly has 100,000 brain cells. A mouse has 5 million. A monkey has 10 billion. A human in comparison has 100 billion brain cells to work with, states Ronald Kotulak in *Inside the Brain*. This huge jump in brain cell capacity, mental ability, and our incredible skill for learning has made humans a breed apart from most of the animal kingdom. Because of this mental capacity, the scientific name for human is *Homo Sapiens* which means Wise Man. This large brain needs data from inside body and from the outside world in order to stay in shape.

Along the path to understanding our search for mental stimulation and creativity, the development of the human brain is where it all starts. The repercussions of this brain have had global significance: Humans have caused extinctions, changed climates, created dams, skyscrapers, highways, cement roads, bridges, cut trees, processed oil, dug for minerals, waged war, created DDT and pesticides, unleashed atomic energy, and performed genetic manipulation, to name only a few.

Who are we? Interestingly enough, we are on the primate genetic line since more than ninety-eight percent of our genes are shared with chimpanzees. Thus, the questions immediately arise: How did we get from there to here? Why do we fill and dominate almost every niche on earth while the rest of our chimpanzee relatives are still swinging through the family tree?

The Brain

Historically, the primate brain was a long time coming. At the beginning of life, the first important step in the evolution of the brain was a cell or part of a cell which eventually became the neuron. Without this neuron, the rest of animal evolution would never have taken place.

The neuron, the basic brain cell, is an octopus-shaped cell on a thick stalk, which is activated by bursts of electricity and units of chemicals called neurotransmitters. These neurons do not only occur in the brain, but are the unit of the nervous system throughout the body. One neuron can connect to hundreds or even thousands of other neurons in the body by branches called dendrites. The electrical pulses sent by neighboring neurons travel in through the arms of these dendrites to give the neuron

Chapter One 8

The Neuron

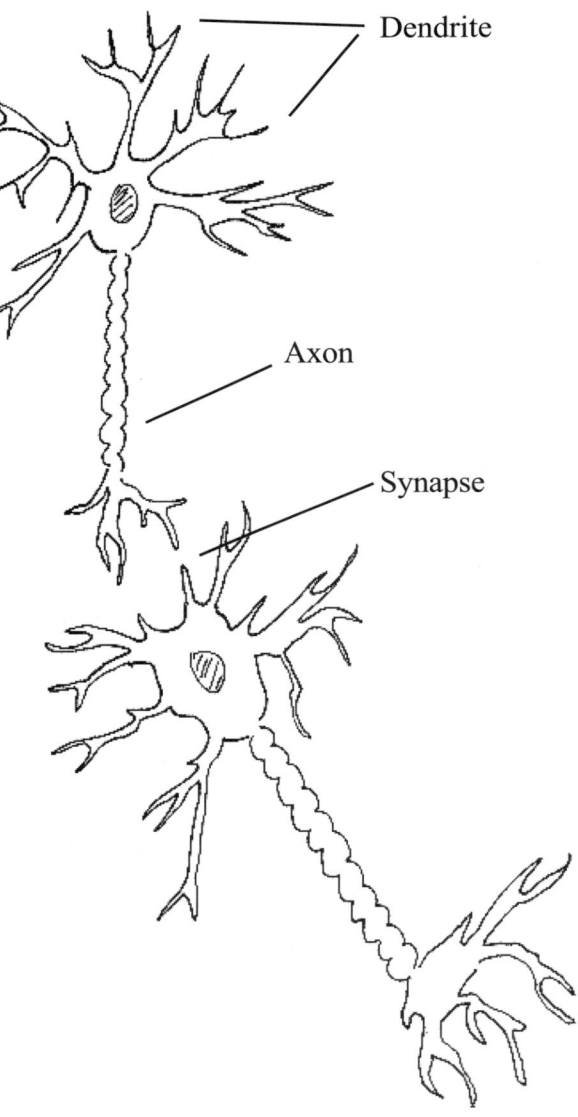

feedback and information from surrounding cells. There are enormous numbers of dendrites in the nervous system to receive incoming data.

The outgoing message line is called the axon, the stalk, which sends electric charges out to the tip of the axon which then activates chemical messengers (neurotransmitters) that span the small gap, called the synapse, between the axon and the receiving dendrite from another neuron. As the electrical energy is translated into chemical energy, it receives a boost in strength. The neuron performs a wide variety of functions. As well as receiving messages, the dendrites store much of memory and perform other important functions of the brain as well. It is the neuron that allows us to receive stimuli from the environment and permits this stimuli to travel to the brain for interpretation.

The second noteworthy event in brain development was the evolution of the so-called reptile brain, a sort of basic brain structure which is in charge of elementary functions such as breathing, heart beat, and all the automatic systems that we take for granted. The simple systems need to be in place before more elaborate systems can be added on, just as the Model T was created before the Mercedes.

Third came the limbic system, the emotional system. The emotional system has a main function which is to initiate those actions and reactions that need to take place instantaneously and cannot be trusted to the slower cognitive thinking system. For instance, evading predators requires an immediate reaction. The quicker the response, the more likely that the human or other animal will survive. Those who are unable to make the quick exit become a predator's dinner and are quickly weeded out of the gene pool.

Another reason for the limbic system is to form the emotional and nurturing bond between the mother and her young from which the emotion of love emanates. Many times, depending on the particular species, the father is included in this system, too. All mammals that raise their young use this bonding system. Mothers (and fathers, depending on the species) and young need to be well bonded, especially in animals like humans who take care of their young for an extended period of time. Human mothers and fathers are both concerned with the teaching of the young, because the baby is born in such an immature condition and needs close to twenty years to learn the complexities of being human. As a result, human feelings of love and bonding are very strong.

All mammals have a developed emotional system. If we are having a bad day, and our dog or other pet tries to comfort us, this comforting is a reasonable interaction between mammals. The pet, especially if it is a mammal, has an emotional system and can tell when we are suffering an emotional crisis and may want to help. Without doubt, it is this shared system that allows the bond between pet and human to develop in the first place.

The fourth significant event in brain evolution is the creation of the neocortex. This thinking apparatus, which evolved to act as a brake to the emotional system, allows for cognitive thought. If the neocortex has time, it can override an emotional response.

The emotional system being first and foremost in the brain, has the ability to evaluate an event and send the whole conscious brain into crisis mode. Interestingly, events that happen in the emotional system need not register in the neocortex. This separation of cognitive thought and emotion demonstrates that the brain is not one unified whole.

In fact, the brain is actually a conglomeration of bits and pieces. During the process of evolution, the brain could not shut down while it was rewired, so any additions and improvements had to be accomplished while the less evolved brain was still operating. One of the ways to complete this task was gene duplication. The old gene kept the current system working while the new gene, a mutated copy of the old gene, tried to change the human in some way. The new mutated gene was acted upon by natural selection; i.e. if it was beneficial, that human survived; if it was detrimental, that human died out. Gene duplication has provided many of the upgrades of the human brain that have taken place in the past and will continue to take place in the future, says John Allman in *Evolving Brains*.

The brain evolved to help us adapt to a world that

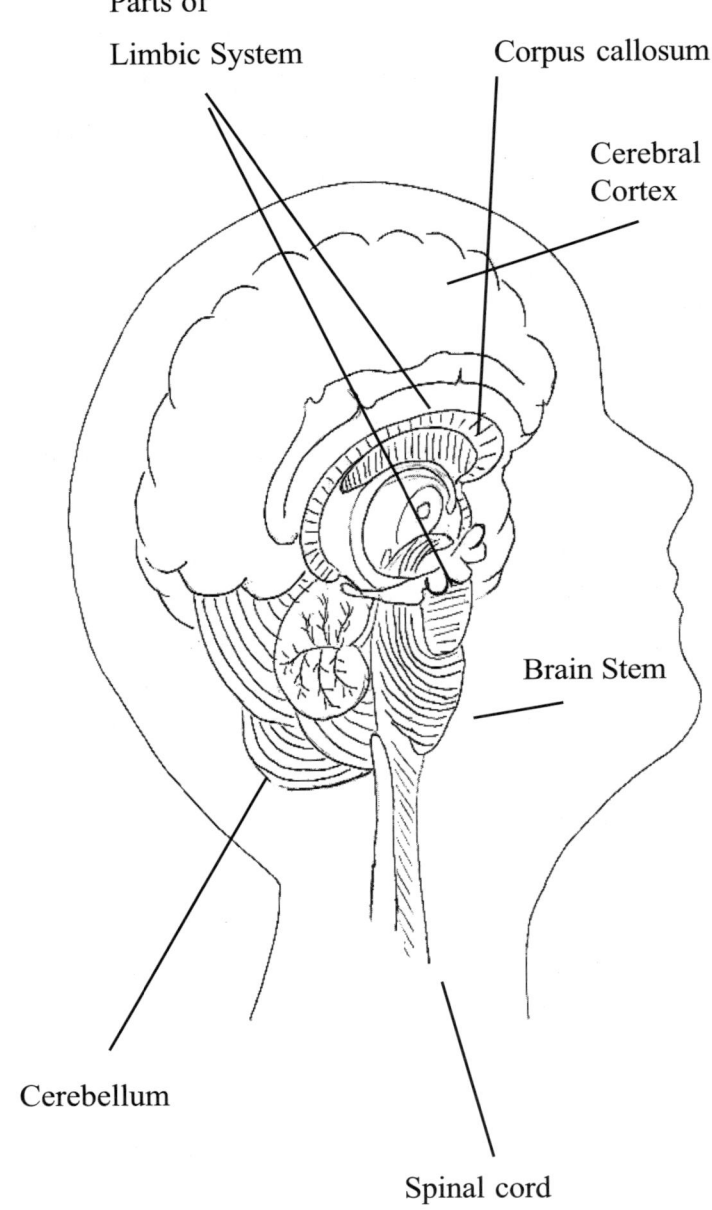

is no longer current. Fortunately or unfortunately, the thinking and learning patterns of our species were developed millions of years ago. For example, living in cities is a relatively recent development. Humans have lived in cities for less than one thousand years and have had agriculture for less than ten thousand years. For more than a million years before that we were recognizably human and living, mostly in Africa, probably as foragers. So the modern city dweller has a brain that was designed for hunting and gathering in small groups on the African savannah, explains Matt Ridley in *The Red Queen.*

The African savannah was an area of green rolling hills, small trees, and wide open spaces abundant with prey and predators. The human thinking patterns designed for this environment, such as noticing new events and reacting quickly, do not effectively coincide with the current supply of chronic dilemmas of modern civilization. We have changed our environment but not our psychological outlook that was adapted to it. We become stressed when we have to deal with long-term problems that are hard to solve.

How did we get from the savannah to the city? There are three main theories of how the human evolved from a primitive being into an advanced species, as mentioned by Elaine Morgan in *The Aquatic Ape.* The first theory, the Savannah Theory says that at some point hominids (early pre-humans) noticed that chimpanzees were doing a better job of living in the trees than they were, so the hominids decided to leave the trees and try their luck on the green, rolling hills of the African savannah.

The savannah was a vastly different place from the tropical jungle for there was no fruit available but herds of tasty wild animals roaming the grasslands. These herds attracted other large, very successful hunters into the neighborhood. The early prehuman had to quickly learn how to cope with these large hunters. Going from a fruit eater, basically vegetarian diet to the meat diet of the savannah and all that it included, was a huge leap for the early prehuman. Many animals could not make such a drastic change.

The complex human brain had many reasons to evolve. In order to compete with other large predators, the necessity to be an efficient hunter with more memory was a primary concern. Enhanced memory let the hunter remember where the prey was and how to successfully catch it. The better hunter required a larger brain which needed more fuel to remain cool. Resting mammals typically expend five to ten times as much energy as do comparably sized reptiles, says Allman. In addition, as humans became more modern, the bigger brains evolved to deal with greater environmental uncertainty that occurred with longer life spans, says Allman.

`The larger brain provided the opportunity for the human to learn all during his entire life span. The arboreal primate had a developed brain, but when the primate hit the ground, he was forced to hit the ground running and the need for a larger brain quickly followed.

Among various other activities, humans use their larger, developed brains to outsmart each other. Living in a society full of smart, manipulative, competitive human predators all looking for dinner, social advantage, and mental stimulation is no easy task. Even today, we spend much of our time using our minds to manipulate, protect ourselves from, and get along with our fellow humans.

The second theory of human development states that many groups of mammals have a member that returned to the sea. The bird family has the penguin, the bovine family has the whale, and possibly the ape family has us. Hence, the human possibly needed to acquire a variety of skills and abilities to adapt to this new environment. The ability to adapt to different environments helped create the flexibility of the human brain.

We have some special characteristics that are shared by water dwellers. One example is that if a person takes a deep breath, and sticks his head in a bowl of cold water making sure that his face, nose, and eyes are fully immersed, after 30 seconds, his heart rate drops 10-25 percent. This trait enabled us to dive better and slowed our oxygen demands when under water. Some scientists, claims Hasseltine in an article "Fear and Evolution" in *Discover Magazine*, believe that the human ability to hold his breath and control oxygen shows that at some time our primate ancestor probably spent as much time in the water as on land.

Elaine Morgan argues that the human primate returned to the water for a million years or so when large parts of northern Africa were under water. In fact, she believes that upright stance may have been water-related; humans may have waded in the water looking for clams, small fish, and snails that could be picked up with the grasping hand in the shallow water. The resulting upright stance freed the hands to manipulate everything from a shellfish dinner to rocks and clubs. The variety of actions brought about by upright stance once again promoted brain expansion.

In addition, during the course of evolution, humans lost the heavy coat of hair that covers most primates and have acquired a fat layer under the skin. This fat layer resembles those of other aquatic or semiaquatic animals such as porpoises, whales, seals, pigs, and hippos.

As a result of this layer, human babies are fat compared to ape babies, which adds to their buoyancy in the water. Thus, human babies take very well to swimming at an early age, hence all the mother and child swim classes that are now offered to take advantage of this fact. Most other ape babies are not attracted to water.

It is important to note that wherever we live, we create swimming pools, both public and private, and gather by the thousands to crowd the local public beaches where we bask and bathe on hot summer days. Not everyone, however, agrees with the theory that humans are semiaquatic.

The third theory of human development deals with neotony, which is demonstrated by an animal that begins to have more success in youthful stages of development and, as a result, the animal spends more and more of its life in immature stages. A perfect example of neotony is the dog, which remains in an eternal puppy state rather than maturing into a full blown wolf. However, the dog was bred by humans to be easier to control and the dog lost not gained intelligence. Since the human infant is born so immature, it gives the human baby longer to learn more information and skills for coping with life.

Matter of fact, neotony may be one of the reasons that Cro-Magnons, modern humans, succeeded and the Neanderthals did not. Neanderthals and Cro-Magnons were two types of humans that were living simultaneously in Europe. The Neanderthals were bigger and heavier and their offspring were presumably more mature at birth, thus depriving the young Neanderthals of the time and the opportunity to learn as much as the young Cro-Magnons. The Cro-Magnons therefore won the day by means of their longer period of learning and greater intelligence.

Thus the different stages of evolution provided humans with more flexibility than most animals, a larger brain in comparison to body weight, upright stance, more complex, grasping hands with opposable thumbs, and more intricate emotions and thinking processes. These characteristics are all prerequisites to preparing the human to be a creative, innovative and adaptive being.

QUESTIONS TO CONSIDER

1. WHAT PROBLEMS ARISE FOR HUMANS LIVING IN LARGE CITIES WHEN THEIR BRAINS DEVELOPED ON THE AFRICAN SAVANNAH?

2. DO YOU THINK HUMANS ARE SEMI-AQUATIC?

3. WHY ARE WE SO DIFFERENT FROM OTHER ANIMALS? OR ARE WE?

Chapter II   THE SENSES

The senses are the means by which we receive data about the world; these sensory systems are intricate and complex. To maximize the accuracy of incoming data, we learn to correctly interpret the information that our senses bring and realize its limitations. In addition to receiving data, the senses are very important to our ability both to appreciate and create art work as we shape and reshape our environment.

Before we can explore the senses, we must talk about consciousness which shouldn't take too long since, unfortunately, no one seems to know exactly what consciousness is. Daniel Drubach in *The Brain Explained* states that consciousness is defined as "a mental state in which we are aware of events taking place within ourselves and our surroundings." Consciousness is the state in which the body is open to receive input from the senses.

Surprisingly, the brain is conscious even during sleep because the brain can still react to loud noises and other stimuli from the environment. If the brain is unconscious, only the automatic processes are working. Consciousness, however, is not the beginning of all. Robert Ornstein, the author of *Evolution of Consciousness*, states that the unconscious knows a fraction before the conscious brain when the conscious is going to precipitate any action. If our subconscious knows we are going to act before our conscious does, then who is running the show? asks Ornstein.

Perception from our environment is an immediate event. We can only perceive stimuli from the environment when the stimulus is actually hitting our senses. Once the stimulus is gone, we have memories but no longer perception. Perception includes both stimuli from the environment by way of the senses and perception of our interior thoughts by way of thinking.

The brain is very plastic. The minds of adults are constantly being changed, remolded, and rewired according to the stimulation that the adult receives and the new material that is constantly entering the brain through the various senses. John Ratey in *User's Guide to the Brain* writes that "it is not an exaggeration to state that after you have an experience, you are not the same person you were before the experience. Experience colors perception."

The brain is ready for action and is always running at a level of minimal neural activity. If each neuron was completely inactive and had to reactivate each time a stimulus came into the environment, reaction time would be dramatically slowed. For this reason, the senses are always firing at low frequency to remain prepared for action and reaction. Ratey gives a great example of what consciousness means to him. He explains that the brain is continually firing small bursts of energy in random patterns, like musicians tuning up for the symphony concert. It is only when the conductor arrives and raises his baton that the symphony starts working together. Consciousness is when the conductor arrives and the whole brain starts working in one great united effort.

However, confusing incidents sometimes happen. There are times where the body receives information below the conscious level, such as in the case where subliminal messages are flashed on a movie screen. The eyes are not fast enough to read the message but the message still registers with the mind. So, in certain instances, the body can receive messages though the senses, but not along the usual path. It seems that there are parts of the brain that kick into action when the normal senses fail. The information goes through the senses but registers in the subconscious mind.

Sometimes background emotions interfere with perception. For instance, stress can cause interruption and reduced efficiency in all the senses because it causes neuron overload much like static on the radio. In this way, overstimulation of the senses, such as fear, anxiety, and depression can hinder our ability to use our senses and our memory. Modern society with all its stresses, has a negative effect on the human body in many instances. To survive, we humans learn to minimize our stresses, especially the continual bombardment of the senses.

In the case where our senses are being affected by internal or external stresses, the data received may be distorted. We must take this distortion into consideration when interpreting incoming data. For example, a person might want to wait until he is not tired or angry to decide whether to accept the new job. A seething mother may want to get a second opinion or wait for a better time to discipline her teenage child.

Not all of our senses are of equal importance. We rely heavily on sight, hearing, and touch. Smell and taste are used to a lesser extent, mainly with our intake of food.

As the senses relate to art, supposedly, we could say that haute cuisine is art for the sense of taste and perfumes and other fragrances are art for the sense of smell. However, in taking art as a whole, taste and smell are not as important. Hearing, touch, and sight are where we concentrate our perception of our environment and our arts.

According to Drubach in *The Brain Explained,* perception is a complex system but only a fraction of the information our body gathers. Our body gathers additional information from the environment and from within ourselves that is not perception because it does not occur at the conscious level. The subconscious gathering of data occurs with the more complex functions that humans perform. For instance, when we walk, we have a knowledge of balance, where things are located in the environment, and where our body is located in the environment but these bits of information do not register with us consciously and are not part of our conscious perception.

Sight

Diane Ackerman, in *Natural History of the Senses*, advises us to look in the mirror and recognize that we have the eyes of a predator. She's right. Our eyes are set in the front of our faces so that we can chase and grab prey as well as swing from branch to branch through the forest canopy like our distant ancestors. Both of these activities, hunting and movement through trees, require good depth perception. From the top of the forest canopy, one bad decision in reaching for a branch and it is a long, potentially fatal fall to the forest floor. Good depth perception was a necessity for a primate.

The eye has had an interesting development. The most primitive eye in early evolutionary history was used by a sea organism to avoid predators and follow sunlight, says John Allman in *Evolving Brains*. Later on, many of the characteristics of our eyes were determined about 55 million years ago by small, nocturnal primate ancestors that moved through the trees at night hunting for insects.

The actual eye works like a camera in that it gathers light and focuses it on the back of the eye called the retina where the impulse is then sent to the brain for interpretation. Thus, it is actually the brain that interprets sight. In brain scans, the brain has six different areas that are activated in visual processing, demonstrating that vision is a complex process. The eye itself further makes many additional compensations for light, shadow, distance, and color change and variation. Human eyes have successfully evolved to compensate for motion. Primate eyes have a special adaptation which stabilizes the retinal image so that it will not be blurred by physical movement, as when the predator is hunting down game or swinging through the trees.

There are drawbacks to having keen eyes in the front of the face. One of the drawbacks is that the primate has no visual defense from the rear and no ability to sense danger coming from behind. Allman theorizes that this lack was probably instrumental in causing primates to become social, so that some member of the group could always be alert to oncoming danger from any direction.

Sight is the most powerful of our senses. The fact that we are tall and upright lets us use our eyes extensively. Because of our height, we can scan the horizon or look at something at our feet. We can see distant and close up. The human is capable of telling the correct size of an object without any other visual cues out to a distance of about three feet. This is the area in which the sight from both our eyes converges, says Allman. After that, the human underestimates the size of the object.

If the human is allowed background cues, he can give the true size of an object out to about 90 feet. Children under eight years old can only estimate size up to 9 feet. Apparently, says Allman, one of the reasons for the slow maturation rate of the human brain is the necessity for experience and feedback for the child to learn distance relationships.

A baby, of course, is preoccupied with studying the environment up close and personal. Everything is tested by sight, taste, and touch. As the child matures, she can look farther away and does not need the close sight that the baby used to test the environment. For this reason, it is normal for adults to lose the clarity of near-vision that they once had as babies.

Once again, idle brain cells will migrate to stronger areas. If one eye becomes considerably weaker than the other, neurons from the weaker eye will be put to work in the stronger eye. For correction, glasses are important to keep both eyes seeing equally with an equal distribution of neurons and may help the brain gather more realistic incoming data.

Ackerman states that abstract thinking may have evolved from the our ability to see so much and then the subsequent need to interpret what was seen. We can see in the distance, so we have time to think over an urgent problem and prepare a response to oncoming danger.

Much of our learning occurs through our eyesight. We read books, observe others' actions, and experiment through trial and error to gain insight and knowledge. However, our sight only gives us a rough approximation of reality at best. Our eye actually sees only a thumbnail size portion of whatever we are looking at, and any other information and any blind spots are filled in by the brain and its knowledge of the outside world. Obviously, our view of the world is flawed. It's amazing that we see so little and think we see so much.

The human eye, of course, has the power to see in color. Humans use three different types of color-detecting cells in the eye: red, blue, and green. On the other hand, fish use four different color-detecting cells and birds have up to seven. Compared to the way that birds and fish see the word, our lives are monochrome, says Matt Ridley in *The Red Queen*. Some other animals only see in black and white, and some insects see phosphorescent colors that we cannot. Women are generally better at seeing color because men have a much greater incidence of color blindness.

Our human primate ancestors gained the ability to see in color in order to differentiate a ripe fruit from the background in the forest canopy. Interestingly enough, in the areas where the primates lived, the color in plants evolved about the same time as color vision in primates. Plants attracted primates to the seeds and fruits so that the primates would disseminate the seeds throughout the area. This relationship between plants and primates is perhaps why the appearance, odor, and taste of fruits and flowers are so attractive to the human, says Allman. We have taken this love of color and made it an important part of our lives as well as our art. People surround themselves in the colors that they enjoy.

Our eyesight has produced interesting effects on our culture. Humans have created art, wall paper, brilliant fabrics, bright clothing and class distinctive clothing, Christmas lights, parks, written music and written books, fire works, haute cuisine, architectural designs, TV, movies, computer, videos; all of these and more because our eyes enjoy seeing novel stimuli. Our delight in our eyesight has had dramatic effects on our society.

We use our eye sight to try to read other humans. At first meeting, we use our eyesight to judge and evaluate each other. We scan each other for pleasantness, danger, interest, attraction, social position, credibility, sophistication, education, and occupation. The data from our sight is influential in the shaping of our relationships, our society, our environment, and our art.

Touch

Touch is one of the most important senses to the developing human. Without touching from fellow humans, a child will never develop into a successful adult.

The receptors for touch, of course, are located in the cells of the skin. Touch is registered when a slight pressure is placed on these skin cells. Since the skin covers the entire body, the sensor for touch is the human's largest sense organ.

Touch enables the newborn to develop normally and to start discovering the world in which she lives and functions. Touch is a form of communication. For example, one baby needed surgery soon after birth. After the surgery, he was given curare, a drug to paralyze him to keep him from tearing out his stitches. When he was paralyzed, his heart beat wildly and only slowed down when his mother rubbed his cheek and his belly. Babies who are caressed and held develop more quickly and are calmer than those who don't. The power of touch is strong.

As well as registering touch, the skin reacts with feelings of pain when something sharp, hot, or abrasive harms the skin. The sense of touch alerts the body to dangers in the environment, as in the immediate danger produced by a spider crawling across the skin.

Touch cells stay calm for everyday events that are not important. For instance, wearing clothes stimulates the touch cells, but the cells do not react because they are accustomed to clothing. As with the other senses, touch cells are clued to react solely to new stimuli in the environment.

According to John Ratey in *User's Guide to the Brain*, Frederick II in the Roman Empire wanted to see what would happen to children without touch and language. He took a number of newborns from their parents and gave them to nurses who fed the babies but were forbidden to touch or talk to them. The babies died before they could talk, thereby showing the importance of touch and language.

A component of touch that we share with the apes is the capacity for tickling, which elicits laughter. "Tickle may be at the root of all play, " writes Provine in *Laughter,* who claims tickling helps parents bond with their young and later helps lovers bond with each other. All parents know the joys of tickling a baby who responds with delight to the slightest touch. Yet, extreme tickling is considered a form of torture as in "tickled to death": Another instance of a stimuli that has a certain threshold for pleasure and beyond that comes discomfort.

Deprivation of touch can cause the death of brain cells. Humans are a social animal and there is no way to get around it. Human babies in the United States are isolated from human touch more than babies in other societies or in primitive tribes who carry their children wherever they go. Our babies are put in strollers, carriers, cribs, play pens and are distant from the mother.

How much people touch each other is cultural. Many Europeans touch, hug, kiss each other more often than Americans do. Ratey believes that cultural touching is important because "cross-cultural studies have demonstrated that societies in which parents show more physical affection toward their infants and children tend to have significantly lower rates of adult violence."

The sense of touch plays a central role in our society. From hugs to the ancient art of massage, touch is a necessity in our lives. The sense of touch allows for the delicate use of our hands and fingers in the production of our arts and other activities.

Hearing

Hearing occurs when the ear picks up fluctuations in air pressure. These fluctuations are then translated through a set of small bones in the inner ear, and sent to the brain to be interpreted as sound. Humans can hear frequencies of sound between 16 to 20,000 cycles per second by way of small hairlike cilia which convert the air motions into electric signals and fire neurons along pathways to the brain. Loud sounds, such as rock music or playing the cymbals, can cause the loss of these hair cells and cause permanent deafness.

Humans have developed, along with many other animals, the ability to pinpoint where a sound is coming from. This is beneficial in tracking down prey or locating danger.

Of course, our ability to hear enables us to have complex languages. We judge each other by the speech we hear. We listen for the speaker's words, intent, state of mind, sincerity, agenda, and emotional state. We also listen to ourselves and try to convey what we really mean without emotional or other distortions.

Mammals developed higher pitched sounds which were inaudible to reptiles and bird predators. In this way, the mother mammal had a direct line of communication between herself and her young that could not be heard by marauding reptile or birdlike predators. However, other mammal predators were still a threat. Hearing in non mammals is limited to less than 10,000 cycles, whereas mammals can hear much higher frequencies, sometimes above 100,000 cycles, says Allman in *Evolving Brains*.

The ear is an amazing organ because it combines "a wide-range sound wave analyzer, an amplification system, a two-way communication system, a relay unit, a multichannel transducer that converts mechanical energy into electrical energy, and a hydraulic balance system," says Ornstein in *Evolution of Consciousness*. All in the space of two cubic centimeters. The ear also has two devices called semicircular canals which enable us to know what direction is up, and how to keep our bodies in equilibrium and balance.

Sometimes we take hearing for granted and fail to notice its uses. For example, in games like Ping Pong, says Ratey in *A User's Guide to the Brain*, much of our ability to return the ball depends on our ability to hear the ball hit the paddle, then predict where it will go, then hear it bounce as it hits. Those who cannot hear as well, cannot play as well.

In *The Conscious Ear* by Alfred Tomatis, he explains that we resonate with each other by means of speaking and singing. Since sound causes the air to vibrate, "to listen to someone playing, singing, or speaking is to let oneself be put into vibration with him or her." In this way, we experience closeness by our ability to hear.

The two ears differ, says Tomatis, in that the right ear receives information slightly faster and measures higher frequencies than the left ear. A person who becomes deaf has serious problems. Deafness affects the ability to speak and sing for the singer can only sing pitches he hears and the speaker needs hearing for intonation patterns.

The ear, like the other senses, learns to tune out repetitive sounds. For instance, the ear does not hear the constant beating of the heart or the sound of the blood rushing through the arteries in the body. The ability to hear begins to decline in old age. Although it seems that older people who live in environments with less loud noise, seem to keep their hearing longer. Perhaps the loss of hearing in old age only occurs in noisy societies.

Hearing has led to the enjoyment of music, language, radio, plays, and other entertainment. Hearing lets humans participate fully in the social aspects of their group. Hearing is a vital part of our lives because it protects us from danger and is so essential to normal functioning that we use hearing aids to prolong this ability when it begins to fade.

QUESTIONS TO CONSIDER

1. DO YOU RECEIVE A VARIETY OF DATA FROM YOUR ENVIRONMENT, INCLUDING INPUT TO SIGHT, HEARING, TASTE, TOUCH, AND SMELL?

2. HOW HAS YOUR RECEPTION OF DATA FROM THE SENSES CHANGED OVER TIME?

3. DO YOU HAVE ONE SENSE THAT SEEMS TO DOMINATE THE OTHERS?

4. THINK OF SEVERAL WAYS THAT YOU COULD IMPROVE THE QUALITY AND VARIETY OF STIMULATION IN YOUR ENVIRONMENT.

5. DOES YOUR HOME ENVIRONMENT PROMOTE THE ENJOYMENT OF THE SENSES?

Chapter III
PROCESSING STIMULI

To understand our search for stimulation, the senses are important as they gather data about the outside world. This incoming data is processed in many ways. The usual path for new stimuli to enter the conscious brain is through the senses into different sites where it is interpreted. Any incoming stimulus goes both to the emotional center of the brain to be evaluated for immediate action then to the center for cognitive thought. It travels to the emotional center first since this center is the older of the two. If the emotional center interprets the stimuli as sufficiently important, it can take over the conscious brain and proceed with an emotional reaction. This quick-reaction path has been beneficial to survival during crises, dangers, and emergencies.

The emotional part of the brain was created and solidified before the reasoning part of the brain so emotions have a different network in the nervous system. Emotions, according to Robert Ornstein in *Evolution of Consciousness*, enter through the limbic system into the cortex. This method of entry allows emotions to avoid cognitive control.

For example, when emotionally charged images appear on TV, this information can enter directly into the brain without going through the regular channels of cognitive thought. This allows ads and other emotionally based TV programming to bombard the brain with messages which thereby enter our minds without our permission or our thoughtful consideration.

Cognitive thought acts as the brake; it can negate the action recommended by the emotions if given enough time. If the cognitive area does not act, the brain goes ahead with the emotional response. Cognitive thought requires time to weigh alternatives to make decisions. However, as the workings of the brain are all complicated and interwoven, the limbic system is involved in memory and learning not solely emotional matters.

In certain events, Ornstein states, the subconscious takes control of our actions. While playing the piano, for instance, the pianist's fingers may go faster than is cognitively possible, thereby showing that this particular skill is under the control of the subconscious. Another example is the professional race car driver who drives too fast for conscious control. At some point, he realizes he is performing a very dangerous action on autopilot.

Love inspires us

Love is very important to creativity and the desire to create art. The intense feelings created by love are channeled into other areas of people's lives and some of these emotions reemerge as art works.

The capacity for love is determined by how much love and what quality of love the baby receives from her mother. If the mother is nurturing and conscientious, the baby will be confident and able to love. If the mother is uncaring or unable to love the child for some reason, it will greatly hamper that child's ability to love when the child gets older. The formative years are important emotionally as well as cognitively.

The child learns about love from his parents and is programmed for mate selection by childhood experience. These early feelings stay with him well into his adult years. When he meets someone as an adult, "The closer a potential mate matches his prototypes, i.e. the patterns he formed as a young child, the more enticed and entranced he will be—the more he will feel that here, at last, with this person, he belongs," says Thomas Lewis in a *General Theory of Love*.

Romantic love and mate selection is vital to the survival of the species; for this reason, nature does not dare place this process under control of our intellect. It becomes an emotional loop which guarantees immediate action. Love certainly colors perception by making people spacey, more docile, and high on serotonin and other hormones. People in love see the world through rose-colored glasses. Love is an emotion with survival value that has the ability to dominate people's thinking and take control of their actions

Chemicals in the brain work to keep the person in love on good terms with the group. Serotonin, one of the hormones involved in love, seems to stabilize the relationship between the person and the group. There is a good example in monkeys: male monkeys who had increased serotonin, became more friendly with the females of the group, and they rose in the power structure because they had more friends on their side.

Love is both chemical and intuitive. Attraction between two people is difficult to explain, because it is the intuitive system that is making the decisions, not the cognitive processes. Something in the intuitive part of our brain recognizes that this certain person fits our ideal prototype, says Lewis, who talks about the stages of love. This is called *attraction.* We are off and running, whether we like it or not.

The next step in the process is *fixation* which is very much like the process of imprinting that occurs between the duck and its mother. When the duck is born, whatever walks by will be followed by the young duck because the duckling imprints on that being as mother. It makes no difference if the being is a mother duck or a human.

Fixation comes in two varieties: benign and malignant. Benign fixation includes the usual fantasies, day dreams, being inattentive to normal life, and being blissfully full of Mother Nature's painkillers, the endorphins. Endorphins, according to Norman Cousins, the author of *Anatomy of an Illness*, are substances much like morphine that occur in the brain and create the body's own anesthesia and relaxation. However, anything that includes high emotions also has a down side. Some people cannot stay in the benign state without starting to wander over into pathological fixation which might include such unpleasant behaviors as stalking, jealousy, and abuse.

The next stage of love is the *reckoning*. We need to determine if the other person shares some version of these same feelings or if we have been floating in a cloud of endorphins for no reason whatsoever; i.e. whether our feelings are reciprocated or not.

Next comes the *leap of faith*. We cannot ever be completely sure that the person we love is the perfect one. So, in love as in any big decision, there is risk. The lover has to be willing to gamble that his beloved is the right one. People occasionally take actions that are not based on any tangible guarantee, love is one of those gambles.

Love is probably responsible for influencing and inspiring more creativity than any other human emotion. It is so strong that it often necessitates expression in one way or another. Creativity and the arts provide a welcome outlet for this strong emotion.

Unfortunately, we cannot direct our emotional lives in the same way we can perform a physical movement, says Lewis. We cannot will ourselves to want the right thing, love the right person or feel happiness after disappointment. Will works in the logical, cognitive part of the brain but not through the emotional system. We simply need to work through the emotional experiences the best that we can.

Since people are social, a person without personal, loving relationships is a desolate being. Throughout history, many artistic types have led rather isolated lives. It may be that the artist needs to be isolated to create and it may be that the isolated person reaches for the arts to feel and communicate on an expanded level. Often the artist tries to speak to the community through his or her art.

Mood

Of course, our mood influences how we interpret data received by the senses and how we think. Moods heighten or weaken the amount of energy, enthusiasm, focus, and positive outlook that we can focus on any one activity. They also become the filter through which we process our incoming stimuli. When we are in a good, positive, energetic mood we see the world as wonderful, ourselves as wonderful and life's events as wonderful. When we are down, we see the world, ourselves, and life as grim and discouraging.

Mood can depend on time of day, on nutrition, and on biological and psychological factors. Most people experience a boost of energy in the morning before noon, and then around two or three o'clock in the afternoon begin to run out of steam, get a short revival of energy in the early evening, then become tired and wind down before bedtime, says Robert Thayer in *The Origin of Everyday Moods*

Since mental and physical systems are all connected, our overall general health can affect our moods. Some serious mood swings are an indication that sickness is on the way. They become red flags that signal the quality of our overall mental and physical health.

What exactly is mood? Thayer defines mood as "background feeling that persists over time." These moods are usually unconscious and not obvious to the individual who is experiencing them. Thayer believes that mood is based on the individual's amount of energy and degree of anxiety. He creates four basic moods on these criteria: calm-energy, calm-tiredness, tense-energy, and tense-tiredness.

• Calm energy is when the person is energetic but not keyed up, simply relaxed.

• Calm tiredness is when the person is just about to go to bed and is calm but tired from the day's activities, but not tense.

- Tense energy is when someone has to accomplish something quickly under a deadline. Some people begin to enjoy the feeling of tense energy and fill up their schedules so that they never have any time to come down. Running on tenseness can be habit forming; there is a high attached to being exhausted and running on empty.

- Tense tiredness is bad news. This mood is the one where the person is tired, tense, on the verge of anger and extremely volatile: a powder keg waiting to blow.

- I would like to add the joyful mood. This is the condition with a lot of creative energy with no immediate tensions. There are times when a person just feels wonderful. Sometimes he or she is doing the right thing, associating with wonderful people, and enjoying the pleasantness of life. Not all is stress and worry.

Color and light can also affect mood. A person's clothing, the color of the walls, and general decor all add to the mood of any particular place. Many people are affected by the lack of sunshine during a long winter in a cold climate and become depressed if they do not receive enough light. These people who suffer from this disorder can be helped by sitting in front of special lights in the winter for mood management.

Humans are always taking their moods into account subconsciously and trying to correct for any imbalances. According to Thayer, the following are the most common solutions that people use to attempt mood management. These solutions or attempted solutions are listed from most effective to least effective:

- **Active Mood Management.** Cognitive activity and exercise is used to induce relaxation and stress management. Men are more likely to engage in exercise than women.

- **Seeking Pleasurable Activities and Distraction.** Pleasant pastimes such as music, humor, or a favorite hobby are used to lighten a mood. Women often go shopping for mood management while men don't care to shop. The arts are helpful here as a means for pleasant activities and a calm distraction.

- **Withdrawal and Avoidance.** In stressful times, the person may want to be left alone to avoid the person or thing that caused the bad mood in the first place. Introverts are much more likely to seek avoidance than extroverts. Introverts are also more likely to do art. Perhaps the introvert who wants to escape from people can find personal release in art projects until the blue mood disappears. In addition, many depressed people who feel down believe that they would not be welcome in a social gathering so they shun others. The arts are useful in this situation in that they take concentrated focus which prevents the person from dwelling on the negative.

- **Social Support, Ventilation, and Gratification.** The person in the bad mood seeks to talk to someone, looks for social support from friends, engages in emotional activity, or looks for gratification. Women, who are much more likely to seek social support than men, are also more likely to engage in ventilation techniques such as crying or screaming, and more likely to eat when depressed. Young people are more likely to vent their frustration in crying and screaming to improve mood. These ventilation techniques do not seem to be extremely successful. Those who ventilate do not seem to be substancially happier than those who don't. However, expressing emotions is better than repressing them.

- **Passive Mood Management.** These activities include watching TV, drinking coffee, smoking, eating, resting. Women are more likely to try passive mood management.

- **Direct Tension Reduction.** These activities include taking drugs, drinking alcohol, and having sex. Men are much more likely to try these methods than women.

Humans have the desire to maximize pleasant moods. When humans feel down, they try to fix the mood and return to an optimistic, energetic state of mind. Unfortunately, this has led to many of the addicitons that we see today. The person may reach for the alcohol or the chocolate chip cookie when he feels down. He then gets a short burst of pleasure which is enough for the body to want to do it again. We can see these unnecessary behaviors and then realize that our brains are merely trying to keep our moods in balance and we really don't need the chocolate chip cookie or the extra beer.

Sensory Deprivation

Periods of sensory deprivation occur in every life and produce mental duress. These periods of duress prevent the normal functioning of the brain and its reception and interpretation of data. Some of the most common examples of deprivation include divorce, the death of a loved one, depression, boring jobs, and old age.

In the case of death and divorce, we have to accept that these people and their input into our lives are gone. Their departure leaves a huge gap which is not easily accepted by the brain, because the input from these people helped to define our reality and with their departure, we must redefine reality for ourselves and readapt to it. We enter a new world.

- ### *Divorce*

Divorce is difficult for many reasons for withdrawing love and caring from a partner is one of the most devastating acts a person can do. Even though the break-up of relatipnships is devastating, the United States is experiencing a state of real transition on the subject of pairing off, marriage, and divorce. In fact, the institution of marriage may be on the verge of disappearing altogether. According to the last census in 2000, the traditional family with one father, one mother, and two children was in the minority. There was an enormous increase in the number of families with a single parent and children and many more people living alone.

More than half the marriages in the US end in divorce. Surely, divorce is traumatic for it causes sensory deprivation and brain alteration. This trauma upsets the balance of the body and leaves it more open to illness. People who lose life partners are at risk. "There are dire consequences to losing a loved one--breaking attachments can affect the immune system and the heart," says Robert Ornstein in *Evolution of Consciousness*. A partner transmits regulatory information that can alter hormone levels, cardiovascular function, sleep rhythms, and immune function, writes Lewis in *A General Theory of Love*.

When a person is left by a lover, the first reaction is protest. The desire to reestablish contact by phone, letter, or email is overpowering. The partner cannot believe that he or she has been left. Just as the baby rat squeaks in distress when mom leaves, so the lover protests strongly when his partner leaves. "The tormented letter that a rejected lover composes turns out to be an updated version of a baby rat's constant peep: the same song, in a slightly lower pitch." says Lewis.

The bereft lover experiences disbelief, shock, withdrawal, depression, anger, lonliness, fear, and many of the same emotions experienced at the death of a loved one.

Granted that relationships are difficult; however, those who think that they can forego them are not being realistic. Adult humans are social animals and cannot function on their own. Human stability depends on the influence of others, for healthy humans are not loners. Processing the different stages of divorce is very much like processing the different stages for the death of a loved one. The difference is that one leaves voluntarily and the other doesn't.

- ***Death***

Another period of sensory deprivation occurs at the death of a loved one. Many people, after completing their years as parents, suddenly find themselves in charge of a dying parent. When a parent dies; they miss their voice, their security, and realize their own mortality. A s Prend says, "When a loved one dies the deepest loss of all, a part of us dies, too, and life will never, ever be the same."

Everyone handles death differently. Linda Richmond in her book *I'd Rather Be Laughing*, describes the tragic death of her 29-year-old son. She bemoans the fact that in the modern United States, people do not want to feel pain or see others in pain. In times of loss, people urge us to buck up that things will be okay. People say that we are strong and we can get through it. The grieving person never gets to admit that he feels distressed and awful. The bereaved is even encouraged to use medications to prevent the feeling of pain.

On the contrary, Richman says that pain is a natural part of the process of accepting someone's death. "I look at it this way: If I didn't love my son, it wouldn't have hurt to lose him. You're supposed to hurt when you lose someone you love. That is just the natural order of things."

There are many strong emotions in reaction to the death of a loved one. These are some other emotions that Prend says the mourner, and the divorced person, have to deal with:

- Anger. How could that person die, how could it happen at this time without giving due warning? Those who get too caught up in the emotion of anger will not heal as quickly as those who are more accepting.

- Guilt. What were the things that were left undone, the words that were left unsaid?

- Pain. Pain and sadness are present at the death of the person who meant so much in the person's life.

- Depression. The mind cannot cope with the stress and shuts down for a while. Some people even develop anxiety attacks or phobias.

- Anxiety. The mourner is afraid that death will happen to yet another member of her family. She might worry more about people when they travel.

- Loneliness. That person might have been the mainstay in another's life. Now he is alone and must start over.

Ashley Prend, in *Transcending Loss,* gives an idea how humans grieve; she lists the basic stages of acceptance of the death of a parent or other loved one. Her three main stages of grief are shock, disorganization, and reconstruction.

Shock is marked by the stark inability to accept that the person's death has really happened. The mourner experiences total disbelief. Some people cry, some become stoic, some might become dizzy or nauseated. The mind can only absorb so much trauma at one time, so it begins to shut down.

Disorganization is the stage which makes a person feel like he and his life are coming apart at the seams. It is very unsettling. It is best to be positive and wait it out. In spite of feelings to the contrary, life will get better with time.

Reconstruction is when the person begins to put his life together again, which requires a conscious effort. Each individual will know when it is time.

Losing one parent is difficult. Losing both parents has repercussions that people might not expect. In Victoria Secunda's book, *Losing Your Parents, Finding Your Self,* she lists some of the complications that arise when both parents die and people find that they are mid-life orphans:

- Seventy-six percent had attachment to siblings change; some closer, some more distant.

- The realization that the parents who were thought of as help in a crisis and sanctuary were gone. This affected relationships with other people.

- For those who are not married, the word "alone" takes on new meaning.

- Some believe that they need to deal with parents' expectations even though the parents are dead.

- If the relationship with the parents was not ideal, there may be feelings of regret or unresolved conflict.

- Women were far more likely to claim that their career choices had been revamped at the death of a parent.

- Many orphaned adults decided it was time to explore the arts to express their creative side, or to enjoy themselves more.

- Women in their grief found friends to help them through; the men had a more difficult time expressing their grief. Many of the men were constrained by the fact that they believed that the expression of grief was not manly.

During these periods of intense emotions, data reception and interpretation is indeed interrupted. A writer who was taking a class in writing experienced writer's block upon the deaths of both her parents. She went into shock and found that her creativity went dormant during her extreme emotinal crises. Fortunately, creativity started to return when the trauma and the loss began to subside about three to four years later. Creativity comes back when the mind and the stamina of the mourner are sufficiently recovered and ready.

It takes at least a year to get over the initial raw feelings, says Prend. The birthdays and holidays have to be dealt with, accepting that the person is gone and will never come back. It takes a while for reality to become your reality. Finally, the bereaved becomes bored and impatient and begins to jump-start the recovery program. He looks for people, adventures, and the means to carry on with his life.

Depression

Depression is one of the states that can arise when the person is deprived of stimulation or on the contrary, when the person is overstimulated, overstressed, and unable to process the situation. The loss of a partner can lead to depression. The mind has been traumatized by loss and grief and semi-shuts down in shock in order to let the mind recuperate and repair.

Depression is a state where the person does not feel like taking action, seeking any adventures, or making any decisions. It is the feeling that, well, nothing is going to work so why bother. Robert Thayer in *Origin of Everyday Moods* defines depression as a compelling, driving, gnawing sense of hopelessness and despair, laced with a heavy mixture of fatigue and anxiety.

It is the fixation on the negative that leads to depression. Some people get tunnel vision whereby the person fixates on something to the point of mental illness. For instance, if the person is fixated on the idea of becoming a millionaire, anything short of that goal is failure and makes the person more depressed because he believes that he has failed. Or if a friend dies, and the grieving person fixates on the idea of this death, he can be headed for depression because in his fixation he does not allow himself the prospect and possibility of seeing and taking positive actions.

The symptoms of grief and depression are similar, the main difference is the length of the period of feeling down. Grief should last about a year while depression, true clinical depression, can last much longer, writes Keith Kramlinger, M.D., in his book *Mayo Clinic on Depression.*

One of the most difficult aspects about depression is that often the person who is depressed actually cannot perceive the levels to which her morale and spirits have sunk. It is the fortunate person who can spot her own depression and then take action to correct it. It is best to tackle depression before it becomes habitual. It can become a mental rut, easy to get into but difficult to escape.

Women, according to Thayer, are about twice as likely to be depressed as men. A possible reason for this is that women tend to think continuously about their problems. This may strengthen rather than lessen the depression. Women are still raised to be culturally more passive which leads to depression. Women are still responsible for domestic and child-raising chores even when working full-time. As a result of depression, women are more likely to eat for consolation. Men are more likely to head for alcohol.

- ***Boring Work***

It is difficult to reach a balance between too much mental stimulation and the lack of it. The only occasion when we reach a perfect balance is when we're dead.

Many boring, repetitious jobs such as assembly line production or early infant childcare, are not very stimulating. These occupations can cause duress to the brain because of simple boredom. Sometimes the mom left at home with a newborn or the man screwing flanges at the conveyor belt may not speak to anyone for a whole day's time. Unfortunately, some researchers think that boring, mentally unchallenging work promotes mental decay in old age.

• *Experiments on Sensory Deprivation*

In the 60s, studies were conducted to determine what happened when people were deprived of any stimulation. There were such experiments as putting a person in a tank of water so that he was floating and could receive no stimulation, or placing the person in a bed and forcing him to remain immobile so that he could not receive any stimulation. One of the most interesting aspects of these experiments was that when they were advertised, many students showed up, but when they understood the details of the experiment, they left. To most humans the thought of being sensorily deprived is a very painful, traumatic event. The avoidance of the experiments demonstrated the drastic nature of being unstimulated. When the human brain receives no stimulation, it creates its own by way of hallucination.

Advanced Years

Old age is a time when the senses start to dim. Some people are deprived of mental stimulation because of this failure or because of serious illness. The lack of input can lead to mental deprivation, sensory deprivation, and social isolation.

Caleb Finch presents the interesting possibility that part of the evolutionary program of early mammals, including humans, was declining function in adulthood or senescence, as quoted by Allman in *Evolving Brains*. Finch says that planned obsolescence for aging humans was an evolutionary adaptation to reduce competition between the young and the old.

Hormones affect the brain as it ages. Humans, and some whales, are the only animals in which the female experiences menopause. This, explains Jared Diamond in *The Third Chimpanzee*, is because childbirth is hard on women due to the size of the newborn. In humans, a 110-pound female produces an 8-pound infant. For the gorilla, a 200-pound mother has a 4-pound infant. For the human female, each successive birth endangers the other children in the family of losing the care and protection of the mother. For this reason, evolution selected in favor of the female who quit giving birth at a certain age. Older females have value as protectors of children both in whales and humans. It was probably the Cro-Magnons, who lived to 60 years, who first experienced menopause because Neanderthals lived only to around 40 years and died too young, says Diamond.

As the senses dim, says Charles Nelson at the University of Minnesota, most people stop taking in new information around the late sixties. After that, they become repositories of information, much like an encyclopedia. The arts can help in all areas of mental deprivation as discussed in Chapter VII.

Memory Enables Stimuli Retention

Memory is necessary to many of our activities because it allows us to remember the data we collect. A person does not realize the importance of memory until in the presence of someone who has lost it. Memory allows us to function as the person we are.

There are two types of memory, says Lewis in a *General Theory of Love.* Explicit memory remembers facts and figures while implicit memory is not available for conscious inspection. Implicit memory is based on intuitive information. The world of love and emotions is based on implicit memory.

Memory is what allows us to consider ideas and actions over time. When a person first processes a stimulus, the stimulus enters first in the short term or working memory of the brain. As it is processed, if the brain thinks it is important or if it becomes habitual, it will go into long term memory to be revived another time.

"Working memory is what makes us most human," says Ratey, in *A User's Guide to the Brain*. "It gives humans the unique ability to predict where we will be and what may happen in the future when we get there. It allows humans to make judgments, anticipate consequences, and take or shirk responsibility."

Long term memory stores memories but not forever. These memories have to be occasionally recalled or they eventually begin to fade. A memory that is never used will be replaced by memories that are more currently useful.

Memory is a much more complex process than previously thought. It was originally believed that memories were stored in some sort of file like photo negatives, in one location, were fairly reliable, and could be pulled up when necessary. With new technology, it has been discovered that memory occurs in little bits and pieces which are scattered around the brain and only come together when the person remembers that particular situation, says Ratey. This diversity is reasonable because a memory can be such a complex entity; it may include sight, smell, hearing, taste, touch which would logically be stored in different places.

In addition, memories are not fixed entities. Every time a person has different experiences, challenges, or emotions, the recalled memories are changed. For example, a memory will be happier if the rememberer is in a joyous mood, and more negative if the rememberer is depressed. Therefore, since details of memories fluctuate on recall, memories are actually not very reliable gauges of the past because they are open to constant revision and reinterpretation depending on what is happening in that person's life. This unreliability has serious consequences for the legal profession where cases are won and lost, depending on the witness's ability to remember. The unreliability and personal variability of memories can easily be demonstrated by getting family together to discuss past events. Family stories and memories are so different depending on each individual's interpretation that it is hard to believe everyone is discussing the same event.

Ratey tells of the experiences of Elizabeth Loftus to show how easy it is to awaken false memories. Loftus, a psychologist at the University of Washington at Seattle, tells about the time that her uncle said that she was present when her mom died.

As a result of this news, she began to have dreams of her mom's death. She could picture the whole scene. There was the crisp, piney smoke from the camp fires, the vision of her mother in her night gown floating face down, the police cars, and the flashing lights that caused her to wake up screaming in the night. A few weeks later, her uncle called to say that he was sorry, he had made a mistake, and she really had not been at the scene of her mother's death after all.

Amazingly, Elizabeth Loftus had completely concocted these false memories from her own mind at her uncle's suggestion since she had never really been present at the scene of her mother's death. Even as a professional, trained psychologist, she was still vulnerable to suggestion. Obviously, we are all suceptible for these sorts of unrealistic memories can be planted fairly easily in almost anyone.

Sleep Solidifies Information

During sleep the brain if far from inactive. According to Daniel Drubach in *The Brain Explained*, the brain consumes more oxygen and glucose during certain stages of sleep than during hours when the person is awake. However, the brain turns off many conscious processes in order to concentrate on subconscious ones. Yet the senses are still receiving data from the outside world.

Sleep may play an important part in putting memories into the brain. Ratey tells about an experiment using a rat who performed certain actions which activated corresponding areas of the brain. Later, when the rat was in deep REM dream sleep, its sleeping mind went through the exact same thought sequences that the awake brain had done when the rat was performing the actions.

Taking sleep into consideration changes the view of learning. The brain accepts a certain amount of optimal data, then during sleep the brain organizes the material before being ready to accept more. Too much material crammed into the brain at one time works as a stressor and prevents the brain from adequately processing the material. An example is the college student who crams a whole term's worth of learning into his head the night before the final exam.

Sleep further plays a role in creativity and problem solving. An artist may ponder a problem or creative concept in the evening and come to a solution in the morning after the brain has had sleep time to work on the problem. Thus, sleep acts as a chance to solve problems that were not solved during the day. Thoughts during the day reach a final arrangement and solution during the night's sleep.

QUESTIONS TO CONSIDER

1. ARE YOU IN TUNE WITH YOUR EMOTIONS?

2. WHAT DO YOU PERSONALLY DO FOR MOOD MANAGEMENT?

3. HAVE YOU EXPERIENCED PROBLEM SOLUTION DURING SLEEP?

4. HAVE YOU EVER EXPERIENCED THE RECOLLECTION OF FALSE MEMORIES?

5. WHAT DO YOU DO TO ENHANCE YOUR MEMORY?

6. HOW DO YOU OVERCOME PERIODS OF SENSORY DEPRIVATION?

Chapter IV
MENTAL STIMULATION, LEARNING, AND THE CHILD

The complex human brain, separating us from most other animals, allows us to have self awareness, language, creativity, and the ability to perform abstract thinking to a greater degree than other animals (except possibly members of the dolphin/whale family.) With this large learning capacity comes the responsibility and burden to constantly feed the brain new information to keep it working at optimum sharpness. This constant quest for mental stimulation often mandates what we do and the goals we set. We are programmed to learn.

The desire to learn is one of the central instincts for a human baby. As soon as a baby enters the world, she begins to analyze and systematize incoming data. Fortunately, along with the wonderful ability to learn, humans enjoy a prolonged childhood which enables them to learn from teachers, parents and other adults who guide them to adulthood. The human baby is born in a very immature condition and takes approximately 20 years to develop into an adult. In past ages, a human was considered an adult at puberty; but with more complex societies, it has taken longer for the young to reach a level of knowledge, experience, and skill that translates into survival.

Stimulation molds the emerging human brain. Neurons and connections between them come and go with mental stimulation. For instance, if the newborn does not hear sound, the baby will lose the capacity to hear because the sound system withers from disuse. The brain cells that were set aside for the sound system, upon noticing the absence of sound, will migrate over to a different part of the brain and enhance that other part. For example, if the baby cannot hear, the baby might develop unusually acute eye sight.

An interesting example of cell migration is the phantom limb. If an arm is amputated, the cells in the brain that once serviced that arm may move to another part of the brain. However, those cells will remember that they were supposed to hurt and will continue to create the sensation of hurting although the limb is missing. Cell migration, cell loss and brain cell rebirth are happening all the time. The brain is far from a static entity.

At birth, the baby is not a blank slate but comes, eager for mental simulation, with many learning aptitudes already in place. Many caretakers and even parents think that all they need to do is leave the newborn in the crib and go about their business. To the contrary, the newborn needs mental stimulation from day one. For instance, a newborn can hear language sounds, see minimal sights, taste, be stimulated by touch and smell, form human attachments, and seek responses from the environment. The newborn may not look like an active learner, but she is soaking it all in and learning an amount so vast that it hardly seems possible. It is extremely vital that brain cells of the newborn receive stimulation. The brain cells and brain connections that do not receive stimulation or connection with some part of the body's functions will die.

By the age of eight months, there are 1,000 trillion connections in the brain, but by age ten, one half of these will die off because they are not hooked up to anything useful or for other reasons not completely understood. So, by age ten, the child has about 500 trillion connections between the cells of the brain which is the permanent condition for the rest of the child's life.

Along the same lines, as one might expect, the evidence shows that the more connections the person has between neurons indicates higher intelligence. The more neural connections the baby manages to create by means of mental stimulation will predict her level of intelligence for the rest of her life.

Genetics, nutrition, luck, care, and the quality and amount of stimuli greatly affect whether the baby will be a rocket scientist or a ditch digger. For this reason, the amount and quality of mental stimulation for the newborn and young child is critical for normal development. Beyond normal development, mental stimulation may hold the key to making a better brain.

However, the mass die-off of brain cells is not entirely due to the cells not being stimulated. Some neurons are believed to die because they are defective. Other neurons may be useful in the formation of the brain and no longer needed after the brain is fully formed and functional, says Charles Nelson, neurologist at the University of Minnesota. There are prohibitory neurons that stop other neurons from firing. Prohibitory neurons can stop an action faster than it can stop itself. These prohibitory neurons may prevent harmful events from taking place in the formation of the new brain.

Because the neural system is still formative, the senses of the newborn do not function at maximum capacity, for a newborn cannot see too well. Both objects that are close and those that are far are blurry, says Ronald Kotulak in his book *Inside the Brain*. Yet items about twelve inches from the face are very clear. This coincidentally happens to be the distance of the mother's face when she holds her baby.

Babies are keenly attracted to faces. If we show them smiling faces, they will look at them for a long time until they get bored. Typically, if we show them the same old smiling faces, they will lose interest. But show a new frowning face, and the babies will once again be attracted to the new stimulus.

Their attraction to faces explains why babies continuously monitor their mothers' faces. If a mother stops looking relaxed, her baby becomes upset and begins to cry in short order. Babies read facial expressions and emotions with unusual acuity because they learn how to react to their environment from the reactions of their mothers and other humans around them.

Babies are attracted to stripes and the edges of things, says Gopnik, in *Scientist in the Crib*, so that they can begin to separate out the different items in the environment. Edges are an easy way to determine where one thing stops and another begins since the edges define the item. Once the edge is defined, the whole item is known.

Newborns know they are human and need to work to be like other humans. Infants enjoy the interaction when someone tickles their feet, smiles or coos at them. When others talk to them, babies enjoy it because they are learning the sounds of the human language, learning what it is that makes a human tick, studying emotions, and determining what they need to know to adapt to their environment. Every society has some type of baby talk that people use automatically when addressing a baby. This modified speech aids in the baby's comprehension and learning experience.

Smells are interesting to newborns. They can identify mother by smell. The baby learns very quickly to identify mother by sound, smell, touch, and the fact that she is the caretaker.

Every time the baby cries, she wants to know that someone is coming to change diapers, feed her, or just provide ordinary stimulation and TLC. Sometimes she even cries just to determine if mom is still there. Manipulation and testing of the environment are the occupation of the newborn.

Since the brain is more fragile than previously thought, the newborn's environment is crucial to the baby's success. Excessively negative stimulation from the environment can cause serious harm to the baby's development. A poor environment is one where the baby is abused, or where the parents are in an abusive relationship. The baby who is upset by cruelty or violence becomes stressed to the point of terror or trauma. In such cases, the brain cells of the newborn start to die from stress. A secure, loving, caring environment with moderate mental stimulation is perfect for the newborn.

It is worth noting that there is a span of mental stimulation that is ultimately advantageous for the learning infant. Too little stimulation deprives the infant of the opportunities to learn and cells die, yet overstimulation also causes undue stress and causes brain cells to die off. Too much stimulation becomes a stressor not a blessing. A delicate balance is required between the two extremes.

TV and Mental Stimulation

The question of adequate stimuli for newborns and young babies becomes especially important in our modern day society where both mothers and fathers are required to work to support the family. Children plunked in front of the TV for baby-sitting purposes when parents are exhausted, or babies neglected and ignored at the day care center may end up with mild mental retardation simply because they did not receive enough stimulation at the early stages of life to ensure normal mental growth.

It is not just cognitive skills that these children never develop but also the budding social skills. "Many researchers believe that communication between humans is the primary ingredient in the development of attachment and social skills," says Robert Ornstein in *Evolution of Consciousness*. Children who are not learning social skills at the right stage in their development have a permanent void that is affecting many different parts of their personalities. "If you fail to learn the proper fundamentals at an early age, then you are in big trouble. You cannot suddenly learn when you haven't first laid down the basic brain wiring," says Rierson, a neurologist, mentioned in Kotulak's book, *Inside the Brain*. Some of these socially deprived children develop into asocial beings in their society with the potential to commit major crimes.

David Walsh in his book *Selling Out America's Children*, believes that our consumerism is denying many of our children the opportunity to receive appropriate mental stimulation and education. TV and video games which attract children are geared to turn a profit without regard to consequences. These games and the media attract children by violence, sex, and humor to emotionally snag them when they are too young to defend themselves. The TV advertisers consider children fair game when they reach the age of three.

Walsh promotes several methods to deal with the screen crisis: Parents can find other suitable activities to do with their children besides TV. The use of TV can be limited to specific times and specific programs. Parents and children can watch TV together so that parents know what programs are being watched and can offer explanations or comments on the content of programs whenever appropriate. The TV can be placed in a secondary position in the house, not in the living room and not in a child's bedroom, in order to promote conversation rather than television viewing.

Granted there are some programs, especially on PBS and other learning channels, that are educational and better for children to watch. These programs are to be encouraged.

In the field of education, times have dramatically changed. Historically, children used to learn by working with their parents and modeling their parents' behavior. At the time of the industrial revolution, people moved to the cities and children were placed in schools which shared the responsibilities of teaching the young.

Less time spent with the family has not been advantageous to the young. The average child spends about 5-10 hours per week in active communication with parents and about 35 hours in front of the TV set; more time is spent in this activity than any other. In fact, television has become the imaginary, unrealistic role model by which children are adjusting themselves to their society.

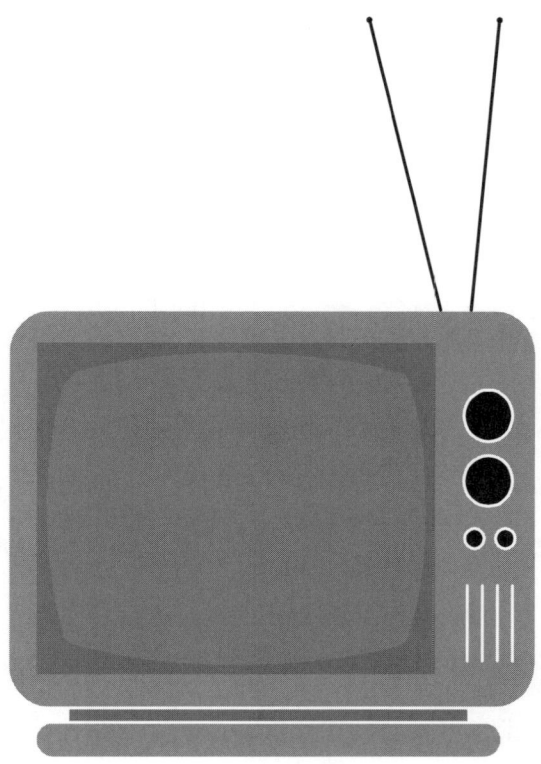

Broadcast TV is especially bad as it goes sensational in order to compete with cable TV and the internet. These are some of the dubious lessons that Walsh believes that children are learning from TV:

- Violence is the solution to life's problems.

- Sex is casual and humorous.

- Material possessions are the key to happiness.

- Rewards without work is the way to live.

- Drugs and alcohol are acceptable.

- Self comes before the good of the family or community.

- Disrespect is a way of life.

- Aggression and disrespect are humorous and attractive.

Many fear problems with learning and TV. Many educators fear that those children who watch too much TV start education with a handicap, according to Jane Healy, Ph. D., in the book *Endangered Minds*. She fears that our society is changing the minds of children by fast-paced, visual stimuli from the screens which further teach children to be physically and mentally passive.

Some children who are overexposed to television and video games can only operate in situations that are broken down into sixty-second sound bytes or can only concentrate on emotionally charged material which includes sex and violence.

In spite of the sedentary life-style requirements of the screens, physical movement is important to mental learning. Energetic people have energetic brains. Unfortunately, in some schools, many PE programs are cut because of school budget deficits. Exercise makes children more content because it pumps endorphins into the brain and creates a sense of calm and well-being. In addition, the physical activity causes better circulation which makes the brain work more efficiently. Humans were not designed to operate without exercise.

The New Brain

Richard Restak in *The New Brain* describes changes that may be taking place in the brain even as you read this. Because of fast paced technology and the media, the brains of many young children seem to be changing toward preferring a fast-paced, multi-tasking mindset. "Our brain literally changes its organization and functioning to accommodate the abundance of stimulation forced on it by the modern world," writes Restak.

Children are evolving to meet the demands of the modern world. "Many personality characteristics we formerly labeled as dysfunctional, such as hyperactivity, impulsiveness, and easy distractibility, are now almost the norm." Restak believes that these characteristics demonstrated by many young students may indicate the future evolution of the brain.

Recent research has further emphasized that the young brain that learns to focus on fast moving data loses the ability to study a topic in depth. Such are the changes that our future will hold.

Language Acquisition

Language is one of the most important milestones in human development. It was with language that humans took an evolutionary leap forward; for language, as the first symbol system, opens the door to other ways of symbolic thinking, such as mathematics, music, and art.

The ability to speak gave early humans a whole new way to look at the world, for language helps to define how we analyze our world. For example, Eskimos have many words for snow while desert dwellers do not. Language partially controls how we think.

Language provides the means for better communication among human groups, thus providing new opportunities for cooperative action such as hunting, social interaction, and enhanced mental stimulation.

The ability to speak was not present throughout primate history, as exemplified by the majority of the primate family who cannot speak. Language is a relatively new process for the primate species and particularly the human animal. "Recruited in less than a million years, nestling separate from the rest of the brain, is a complex of new talents involving language and symbol making," says Ornstein, author of *Evolution of Consciousness*. These new talents are actually a minor part of the brain. As total brain operations go, language, perception, and intelligence make up only about 1-2 percent of the working thoughts that occur in the brain, says Ornstein. In fact, the odds are good that the language centers in our brain were built out of older brain systems that were not originally designed to process language, says Elizabeth Bates of the University of California at San Diego.

However language evolved, it had immediate and profound effects: vocal communication in the group enhanced shared information. As a result, primitive language in early humans helped family bonding and the finding of food. Language magnified the scope of the adult's teaching to the young. Learning language may actually have accelerated the growth of dendrites and aided in the functional maturation of the brain, says Allman in *Evolving Brains*. Language appears to be centered in the cerebral cortex, in the center for cognitive functions, and in adults, most of the language is stored in the left hemisphere of the brain.

The production of sounds is constant in the human from the first cry to the last breath. Without communication between child and caretaker, the baby's development is impaired. Many problems arise in babies who lack affection, care, and family interaction. Without this social support, the baby can become sick, suffer, and have permanent language impairment, states Benedict de Boysson-Bardies, author of *How Language Comes to Children*.

Even though the capacity for language is in place, the baby must work hard to learn the different parts of the language, such as the phonological or sound system. Inside the pregnant mother, in the watery environment which readily conducts sound, the baby hears the sounds of the language she will speak even before she is born. She begins to isolate the patterns and sounds of this language. In just a few months, she will start practicing the sound inventory of her language and she will be able to tell if you are speaking her native language or a foreign one.

The newborn watches intently as any adult or older child makes any sounds. Shortly thereafter, the baby starts to diligently practice these sounds. At birth, every baby is universal, that is, she can produce any sounds or hear any sounds made by humans. By the time the baby is 18 months old, she has become a product of her culture. The toddler will know that the sound system of English has no relationship to the sound system of Chinese, for example. After that, she can only hear and reproduce the sounds of her own specific language, unless she grows up in a bilingual atmosphere.

Language acquisition is a complex skill that takes years to complete. Boysson-Bardies reminds us that the muscles involved in speaking are extremely complex. If we walk into a room and say "Hello, nice weather today," the speech rhythm moves at fifteen sounds a second, and the sound production requires the use of more than 100 muscles. Obviously, the child needs several years before he can control these muscles in a coordinated effort to speak the language well and comfortably.

Boysson-Bardies states that babies process speech in the first two years of life using a dual system: an analytical form of phonetic processing that determines phonemes or what sounds carry meaning in the language, and a more global process that learns to handle words. These first two years set the pattern and the basis for the rest of the language career for that child. Setting the foundation for language use is one of the child's main tasks.

The capacity for language is a human genetic trait, but it is not a free gift. The child will not automatically learn the language into which he is born, but must work hard to internalize the sounds, rules, sequences, intonation patterns, pitch patterns, nuances, and all the other vital parts of the language. From listening to others, the child puts together the grammar of his language.

Learning language and social skills is a stage in the development of the child that cannot be skipped. Children usually start to speak about one year after birth. Boysson-Bardies mentions the three stages that a child must go through in his book, *How Language Comes to Children*.

First, children must be able to organize sensory information and learn to distinguish sounds that are linguistically meaningful to that specific language. Second, the child must learn to segment the language and categorize it, and organize it according to its semantic values. The child must then learn which are the units of the language. To the listener, language comes in one nonstop stream of sound. It is up to the child to determine what are the segments in the stream that carry meaning. Third, children must realize that language is meant to produce meaningful interchanges between people. The child must ultimately be able to recognize the meaning that is being transferred from one human to another.

Not only does the child need to learn the linguistic patterns of the language but the child must learn the body language and other non linguistic communication elements that are native and necessary to that specific language and culture. Extra-linguistic communication can include such things as hugs, gestures, body movements, looks, postures, eye movements and smiles.

The vocal tract of the speaking adult includes the mouth which is horizontal and then proceeds to the back of the throat where it makes a right angle turn and heads down the throat in a perpendicular manner. One of the reasons that toddlers cannot speak properly is that the mouth of the infant proceeds back to the throat where it makes a slanted descent and does not form a right angle. The right angle in the adult allows for better stoppage of the air flow and better speech, whereas the slanted angle of the infant is not formed enough to permit correct air stoppage. By five months, infants have the right angle in the back of the throat. However, there is not control of all the articulators, including the lips and the tongue, until around the age of five.

The phonological system or sound system is complex; infants must realize that sounds are different in different vocal environments. For instance, the (p) in purchase is acoustically very different from the (p) in stop. They must realize that sounds vary from person to person, or place to place.

The vowel system of English is very complex. Each vowel in English has a short sound, a long sound, and an unaccented sound. For instance, 'cab' has the short vowel sound of 'a'. The word 'lake' demonstrates the long vowel sound, while the word 'about' demonstrates the unaccented sound of the vowel. Of course, there are always exceptions like the 'a' in father. Language is a very complex skill to learn. In a language like Spanish, the vowels are quite constant and lack the difficulty found in the English vowel system.

The baby needs to hear many different speakers of the language to learn which variations make a difference and which don't. The baby must accept that all speakers are slightly different in their pronunciation, their word choice, and their speech patterns, i.e. that language as well as identifying the group also identifies the individual. Over time, the baby will learn which variations are acceptable and which are not.

Since the average English speaker knows more than 75,000 words, it is obvious that the newborn needs to quickly start learning the sound inventory of the language in order to learn these words. The baby begins by practicing the sound inventory of the English language over and over again. A lot of the skill that a child will develop in language depends on the amount and sort of language that the child is exposed to from birth. "Children in white-collar families hear 2100 words per hour on an average day, " says Kotulak. Children get an advantage from being in environments where more language is being spoken.

The baby needs to hear others speaking, needs to hear simplified baby talk, needs to hear adults reading, and needs to see small books with pictures. Around the age of five or six, the child will start reading books with fewer pictures. Hearing reading, especially without pictures, gives the child an opportunity to hear new vocabulary used in different situations, a variety of utterances of the language, and enables the child to use her imagination to visualize pictures to go with the language.

When the pictures are provided, the child uses less imagination. However, by the time the child enjoys stories without pictures, she may well be reading books by herself. From her individual language experience, she will put together the complexities of her own language. Since she has unique experiences, her language will also be unique and individual.

Language Acquisition Schedule by Boysson-Bardies in *How Language Comes to Children.*

- *Before Birth*: The baby in utero reacts to voice, sounds, learns mother's voice.

- *Birth to One Month*: The baby works on speech contrasts, prefers mother's voice, recognizes native language, notices sound contour and rhythm of language.

- *One to Five Months:* Child recognizes sounds categories, syllables, intonation patterns.

- *Five to Seven Months:* The child prefers the mother's language, categorizes vowels, sound of sentence structure.

- **Eight to Ten Months:** the baby notices the endings of sentences and phrases, stress patterns and the rules of sounds coming together, beginning of comprehension of words in context.

- **Ten to Twelve Months:** The baby notices word boundaries, knows words without context, knows about thirty words in context, learns words by association of referents.

- **Twelve to Sixteen Months:** The child knows 100 to 150 words, has an understanding of simple sentences.

- **Sixteen to Twenty Months:** The child understands 200 words, can categorize words, understands relationships, sharp rise in vocabulary.

- **Twenty to Twenty-four months:** Child begins to understand word order, gender and number.

Early Childhood and the School

Children learn most of what they need to know before the age of three or at least, they begin to create the capacities for all the learning that will take place in later years. This has tremendous ramifications for the present in our school system. If school starts at five years old as is currently the standard in the United States, the opportunity has already been missed to ensure that the child receives maximum stimulation to guarantee that the child has all systems in place for normal human development, normal learning patterns, normal communication and survival skills. Parents need to see that their children get into preschool programs.

As well as the preschool experience, Children need to experience creative play. Play, says Ratey in *A User's Guide to the Brain*, with its motor abilities and movement skills help the learning of children and social relationships. Researchers are discovering in a number of species that "motor play is almost as important as food and sleep."

Diet is vital for successful brain function in children. Ward Dean in *Smart Drugs II* cites a study performed by Dr. Schoenthaler on over 400 of the most violent teenagers imprisoned in the California Youth Authority. These inmates were given vitamins. Schoenthaler reports that the group of adolescents who received vitamins had an immediate 50 percent reduction in violence. They also had reductions in hyperactivity, insubordination, fighting, truancy, assault, and battery.

Many parent groups are beginning to react against the idea of soda pop and non-nutritive snack foods that are present in most schools in vending machines. Many think that the banning of poor nutrition at the schools would be one way to promote better learning.

In some classes, more than 50 percent of the children take Ritalin for ADHD or attention deficit disorder. Some wonder if this is for the benefit of the students or for the benefit of the teacher who has too many students to handle. Jane Healy, in *Endangered Minds* questions whether we are not drugging the bright kids that are zooming around the class because they are bored while the apathetic, passive ones are accepted.

Our present school system believes that one size fits all. Every child will be happy and mentally challenged in a huge classroom where everyone is supposed to learn at the same rate, have the same interests, profit by using the same material, and learn by the same method. Healy says that it may be time to individualize our school system. Theoretically, this would be great, but no one quite knows how to do it. Not to mention that serious budget problems often prevent innovation in schools from ever taking place.

Howard Gardner in his book *Multiple Intelligences* promotes a teaching method with a pluralistic view of the mind where each child has some of six basic intelligences. The six basic intelligences are (1) linguistic intelligence, (2) logical/mathematical intelligence, (3) spatial intelligence, (4) musical intelligence, (5) bodily/kinesthetic intelligence and (6) interpersonal intelligence. Ideally, the child would be tested and her strengths encouraged.

Most educators realize that students are strong in some areas and weaker in others. The traditional unified theory of intelligence expects a person to be either good or bad at everything and does not allow for strengths and weaknesses.

Gardner believes that IQ tests only test the logical/mathematical intelligence and the linguistic intelligence. Children who are gifted in different areas will get low scores. Our society seems to test in favor of the logical intelligence while placing high value on sports figures, actors, artists, and musicians who do not necessarily excel at logical thinking.

Gardner describes different stages of learning. Young children are eager to try new things. To take advantage of their enthusiasm for learning, young children and preschoolers should be given a variety of experiences and opportunities so that they can get a taste of what is available in their society. Surprisingly, some children in this group may even develop a life-long attraction to a particular field, especially the fields of music and mathematics.

During the elementary school years, students need to learn the basics of symbolic systems and notational systems, such as language, writing, music, and math. This stage needs to be more structured than the preschool stage.

In the adolescent years, the student needs to make a career choice. The student should be carefully guided into the area that is the best fit for his or her strengths.

On the other hand, we would hope that the selection process would not become too programmed so that a student with several strengths could choose his own course. Many people have entered fields where they were not expected to excel. For instance, Eistein flunked chemistry but successfully went on to excel in science.

Now and in the future, it will become necessary to add other kinds of intelligence as the world changes. We need people with environmental intelligence, those with the ability to live in harmony with the planet. Many young people today have high-tech intelligence where they seem to have a prized, uncanny ability to work on and understand computers. Possibly these high-tech skills stem from the logic/mathematics intelligence. At the moment, these students are in high demand.

Children and Art

There are many stages that young people go through before they become seriously interested in art. Many children have a real affinity for the arts and they are not self-conscious about it while they are young. Childhood is a great time for experimentation in the arts because it is then that children often become seriously interested. Howard Gardner in *The Arts and Human Development* discusses art and the young child. He says that at the age of 5-7, universal artistic tendencies may be noticed. Similar drawing schemes, story types, musical patterns emerge in diverse culture and social groups. At this age, children are universally highly creative.

During the ages 7-11, called the latency period, artistic expression continues for most children. Children still draw, hum, compose, rhyme without self-consciousness. This period is critical for the development of the future artist who must develop enough skill and satisfaction at this time to spur her on to future art work.

At the ages 10-14, the budding artist reaches a critical period in adolescence. The decision is made that she either gives up art or decides that art is part of her life.

From an appreciation of rule systems, of relationships between people, of the intracasies of interpersonal behavior, the artist begins to communicate personally and symbolically in art. The budding artist needs encouragement to survive. Without it, the artist will not develop.

What can parents do to promote interaction, art, and creativity with their children?

Many parents wonder how to compensate for the problem of social isolation their children experience with two working parents and the children at day care. Or, the children may be left alone after school without supervision. Here are some suggestions that might prove helpful in encouraging creativity and social interaction for children and provide beneficial mental stimulation:

- Parents can provide their children with varied, positive, interesting mental stimulation. The more experiences a child has, the more his or her brain adapts to new information. The new information provides the framework on which even more varied and complex experiences will rest in the future. To promote the arts, parents can insure that their children receive exposure to the different arts, have a variety of artistic experiences, and the opportunity to be creative.

- Parents can involve their children in interesting conversations. The development of language skills is one of the hallmarks of the modern human. Any lack in these language skills leaves children at a tremendous disadvantage.

- Parents can let their children safely explore and experience the world in which they live. A child's life's work is to become an independent being. The necessity to experiment in a safe manner is crucial to the independent thinking and action of the child.

- Parents can read to their children from books without pictures so that their children create their own visualizations and illustrations in their minds. The ability to visualize and imagine is a key to creative thinking.

- Parents can encourage children to notice interrelations between things; for instance how our actions influence the environment or how two friends react to each other socially. The ability to see cause and effect is a major ingredient in solving problems--cognitive, social, and personal.

- Parents help their children tremendously if they can provide a good home atmosphere, preferably one with both parents being present. Children need role models of both male and female parents. They also need the input and feedback that both the father and the mother provide. They need the security of a reliable family unit.

- Parents should beware of the daycare center that may not be giving the child, especially the young baby, all the stimulation that the child needs in order to function normally within the society. Successful parents pay close attention to caregivers.

- Children need to know themselves. They need to experience time alone as well as spending time with others in a social setting. Writing, art and other creative projects let children get to know themselves. They need to amuse themselves, make their own decisions and yet be guided by the parent.

QUESTIONS TO CONSIDER

1. DOES YOUR CHILD OR GRANDCHILD GET DIRECT CONTACT WITH AN ADULT FOR LANGUAGE AND READING DAILY?

2. IS YOUR CHILD SPENDING MORE THAN ONE HOUR PER DAY IN FRONT OF THE TV OR OTHER SCREEN?

3. DOES YOUR CHILD GET PLENTY OF GOOD NUTRITION AND EXERCISE?

4. DOES YOUR CHILD GET A VARIETY OF NEW, STIMULATING ACITIVITIES DAILY?

5. DOES THE FAMILY PARTICIPATE IN ADVENTURES TOGETHER?

6. ARE YOU AND YOUR CHILD ABLE TO ENJOY THE BENEFITS AND SOCIABILITY OF AN EXTENDED FAMILY?

Chapter V
CREATIVITY

What exactly happens in the creative process is hard to determine because creativity is different for each person and each medium of art or other area of creativity. Further, creativity is something that the creative person does, not something he or she talks about; for much of creativity originates in the limbic (emotional) system of the brain and is not available to the logic that our neocortex (thought processes) understand, writes Thomas Lewis in *A General Theory of Love.* If creativity happens in a center that is not hooked up to our language system, perhaps these ideas cannot be put into words by the brain.

Creativity works with the mind at a subconscious level, for often the creative idea will come to the artist or thinker during sleep and suddenly the idea is there in the morning. Or, the creative person may be working on something without success for a long period, then suddenly the answer arrives. For this reason, people cannot always explain why they did a specific work of art, why they created the new scientific theory, or put together the new mechanical invention.

The creative process takes advantage of the fact that the brain works as a montage and jumps from one association to the next; it does not operate in a linear fashion, says Restak in *Mozart's Brain and the Fighter Pilot.*

Arthur Rothenberg from Harvard believes that creative people in literature, music, science, and math mix and superimpose ideas from different spatial and temporal dimensions into their work. Creative people have a variety of ways to look at any one problem. For instance, Einstein defined energy as mass times the speed of light squared, which was a novel way of looking at the relationship between light, mass, and energy.

Since creativity requires the ability to look at the possibilities in a new way, creativity is individual. This individuality was reported by Howard Gardner in *Arts and Human Development* who tells of an experiment where composers were given a set of poems to put to music. The different methods each composer used to begin and to accomplish the goals were extremely varied.

Though the process of creativity is hard to pin down, Howard Gardner in *The Arts and Human Development,* relates the four generally accepted stages of the creative process:

- **Preparation** is where the ideas are born. During this stage, the artist or inventor is identifying what exactly the project is that he or she wants to begin.

- **Incubation** is where the mind is working over these ideas and looking for possibilities. Every project in art or other creative pursuit takes a certain amount of mental consideration to make the ideas consolidate into a project that the artist or scientist really has a long-term desire to accomplish.

- **Illumination** is the "Aha" when the creator envisions an idea that begins to take form and cries out to become a work of art, book, invention, or new idea. After careful consideration, the creative person finally visualizes what it is that he or she wants to produce.

- **Verification** is when the general plan of action is checked over because the artist is starting the work. The process of checking on the project can proceed during the production as well, so that the project takes different shape and modifies as it progresses.

Creativity occurs in different parts of the brain. "As a rule, creative individuals are 'in touch' with their feelings and express them through their creative productions," says Richard Restak in *Modular Brains*. Restak says creativity requires enriched communication between the two hemispheres of the brain. Restak quotes Joseph Bogen of UCLA as saying that not only does creativity require considerable cooperation between the two hemispheres of the brain but may even require a partial ability of each hemisphere to work independently, "whereby one hemisphere may for a time independently engage in creative production outside of immediate conscious awareness."

Restak states that a high degree of response in the cortex of the brain in reaction to people and events demonstrates the creative person. Since introverts show more cortical response to events and people, it is easier for introverted people to be creative.

Betty Edwards in *Drawing on the Right Side of the Brain* believes that most drawing is done on the right side of the brain. She says that the left side of the brain is analytical, linguistic, linear and slow. The left side of the brain guides the artist to see expectations not necessarily what is there.

In order to really see what is there, the artist must use the right side of the brain which quickly see things as a whole, a gestalt. The right side of the brain, according to Edwards, allows the artist to see artistically.

In the drawing on page 93, the artist flips back and forth between the two ways of looking, says Edwards. If one looks at the linear lines, one sees two profiles, an example of left brain looking. If one sees the whole, the vase, one is enjoying the skills of the right brain as it puts the whole unit together for a total effect.

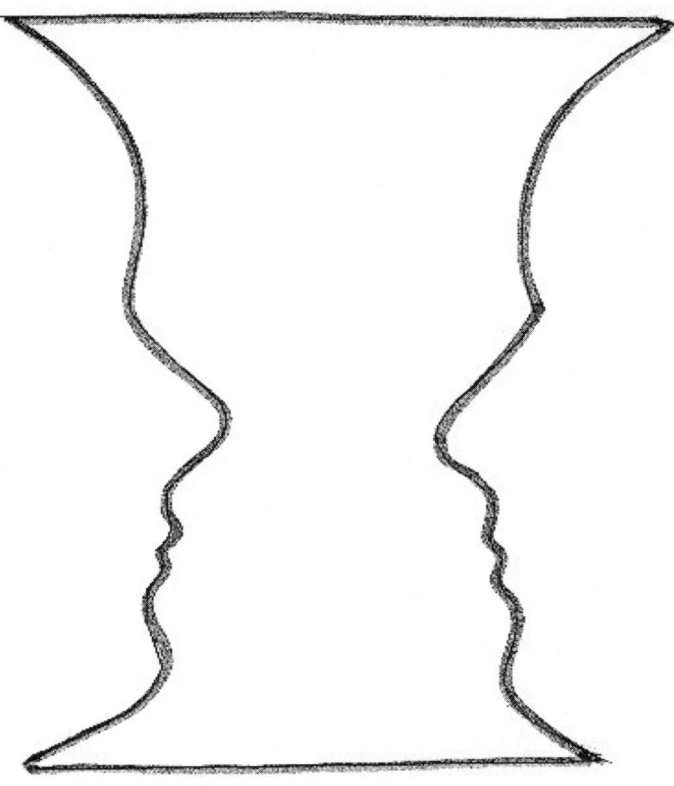

For the creative person, creativity does not remain the same throughout life; it evolves over time. Restak gives the example of the painter Pablo Picasso who started out as a classical artistic and then created cubism and other extraordinary variations of his creativity and art.

Creativity is tenuous. There are no guarantees. Sometimes the creative person simply begins and sees what will develop. Those who dabble in creativity must be brave, willing to take risks, and flexible.

An art project may be more than visualized as the medium begins to take on a life of its own. The artist may decide that the variation he has is better than the one he envisoned. Sometimes the creative person is just as stunned as the observer as to what transpires. On the other hand, the creative person may put in long hours trying to achieve the desired results. After all is said and done, the art work may fail to meet expectations. The outcome may be mediocre or even a disappointment.

There is an interesting phenomenon associated with creating which I call the *"euphoria of creation."* The artist personally takes chaos and turns it into order, a work of beauty and an expression of the self of the artist is born. The resulting art is one of a kind: unique. No one has ever done exactly what this artist has done. The artist feels a tremendous sense of power and satisfaction.

However, the euphoria of creation clouds the artist's ability to judge his work and see defects. Often the artist has to wait days, weeks, even months before he can really look at his work impartially and decide whether it is successful or not. Yet some art works are so immensely satisfying that the artist knows immediately that he has achieved his goal, whereas some works that seem wonderful at the moment of creation do not satisfy a year later.

Oddly enough, formal education may thwart rather than promote the development of the artist. Some fairly talented individuals who attend colleges to study their art are soon cured of their desire to create. At the end of the four years, the students never do another piece of creative art. Perhaps the student, in order to get a good grade, had to give up some of her own personality and self expression in order to please the professor who graded her. This giving up of personal expression to please another is the beginning of the end for creativity.

QUESTIONS TO CONSIDER

1. ARE YOU CREATIVE? IN WHAT WAY?

2. UNDER WHAT CONDITIONS ARE YOU MOST CREATIVE?

3. IN WHAT FIELD DO YOU CREATE?

4. HOW DO YOU FEEL AFTER CREATING SOMETHING UNIQUE? HAVE YOU EVER EXPERIENCED THE EUPHORIA OF CREATION?

5. HOW DO OTHERS RESPOND TO YOUR CREATIVITY?

Chapter VI

THE ARTS AND THE FOUR STAGES OF LIFE

Our ability to learn and create is a continuum that covers our total life span. We have the greatest opportunity to create in youth and in middle age. As young parents and workers, we are too busy. There are four separate stages; each with different lessons to learn. These stages are not carved in stone but are flexible and individual. Some stages may occur earlier or later, be skipped by some or prolonged by others depending on each person's unique life. As a result, our participation in the arts varies with time.

The first stage is the *Student*. This stage begins at birth and is most pronounced until the age of about twenty where it dwindles in intensity but can remain active for years, depending on the individual. We are obviously wired to learn; it defines humanity.

Our brain is formed by our unique genetics, chemistry, and life experiences. No one has ever been like us or ever will be. We are ourselves and begin by learning about the environment; what is harmful and what is not. We learn how to get along with parents, siblings and peers as we shape our social network. In turn, we measure ourselves against the rest of our peer group to determine where we stand in relation to our community. We begin speaking, developing our senses and motor skills, learning life skills, compensating for our weakness and maximizing our strengths.

Because of our differing compensations for our strengths, weaknesses, and different life experiences; we all experience different realities. Within this reality, to appreciate creativity, we need to be exposed to art and creative people as much as possible. We need to begin simple art projects, see if we have any interest or aptitude for art, and receive encouragement where warranted.

Many people who grow to become outstanding artists have early exposure to creative people, enriched environments, and creativity; for artists begin their love of art at an early age. Our early years set the stage for lifelong learning and what we can return to later in our lives. As children, we work hard to set the foundation for the skills we need to function in the adult world. Often, in later years, we return to skills we started in childhood.

The second stage is *Parent, Spouse,* and *Worker.* This stage roughly extends from age twenty to fifty. During this period we learn to love. As a student, we receive love from our parents, but in stage two we learn to give love to our spouse and children. Love is the glue that holds the human family together long enough to raise the children. We have to keep our families together for approximately twenty years, until society says that our children are mature enough to go it alone.

During this second stage, we work the hardest in our lives. We are young enough to have sufficient energy to carry the burden of stress required by this demanding period. We are working the hardest at our jobs to bring in money to keep a household going and to raise our children. We struggle to keep a roof over their heads, learning in their brains, love in their hearts, and good nutrition in their bellies. Needless to say, this period is often exhausting for parents and a trial for kids, but somehow most of us manage to pull through.

Many young adults are now furthering their education and job training while working and raising a family. The total of these tasks combined can lead to high levels of stress on the relationship between mother and father and therefore on the whole family.

Keeping the home running smoothly, taking care of everyone's individual needs as well as the family as a whole, and financing the whole system are some of the most difficult lessons that we learn. We gather many skills: how to manage people, how to manage finances, how to earn money, how to get along as a unit, and how to solve problems as they arise. We learn how to handle stress, anger, bickering, exhaustion, and how to be mediator and negotiator between all and differing elements that cause conflict in a family. We learn to let everyone participate in individual activities but then we all periodically draw together as a family. We learn to cope with all the different parenting skills that our children lead us through, such as how to encourage, praise, train, and reprimand. And sometimes, how to carry on as parents when our hearts are breaking.

At this stage, art and creativity are often placed on the back burner for the typical working adult has little time, energy, or money to spend on the arts. This is a shame because it is through the adult's artistic projects that children can acquire a love of the arts and its place in the life of the family, the individual and the community.

At the end of this stage, children leave the nest. In spite of all plans and preparation to the contrary, children leave a big hole when they're gone. We, parents readapt to being a couple without children in the home. On one hand, we heave a huge sigh of relief but, on the other hand, we miss their energy, vitality and commotion. We ask ourselves, now what?

This leads into stage three: the *Seeker*. This period reaches roughly from fifty to seventy-five. The children are gone and all is quiet. We begin to ponder life's questions: What do we really want to do with our lives? Why are we here? How can we leave our footprints on the sands of time? What direction do we feel we were meant to go?

Suddenly, we find we have time to climb the hills we never had the time to scale before. We begin to seek what we lack or that part of ourselves we abandoned to raise our families. It is a time, once again, to try new things, sample the unique fare that life serves up.

I believe that our society should have a huge ceremony at this time. One part of the ceremony honors the young adult who has successfully grown up without killing anyone, getting on drugs, or flunking out of school. The other part of the ceremony honors the parents who have successfully raised the young adult without killing anyone, getting on drugs, committing abuse. Parents who have given their children the values and skills for success in the adult world deserve acknowledgment.

At this stage, the seeker may find that he or she is looking for more expression and more ways to be personally creative. While the tired parent and worker sought other outlets that were more relaxing, the seeker looks for a more unified way to interact with the environment. He wants to be heard and to express himself in his community and his world. Many are tired of the quest for money and look to more spiritual or creative goals.

It is around this time that parents die. When the

seeker looks around, he sees that the previous generation and its elders are gone. It is an eye-opener. He is hit with the reality that life is truly finite. He begins to urgently ask the questions: Is this all? What do I really want to do in the few, precious years that I have left?

It is during these years that people go through hormonal changes. At this time, they possibly get divorced, have career changes, become retired, try to adapt to an older version of their body, and generally take stock of their lives and see if there are any changes they would like to make before they head into the veteran years. They pursue change and that part of their lives that they have not experienced thus far. And finally, the seekers have to admit to being middle aged.

The final stage of our lives is the *Veteran*. This period extends from seventy-five until the end. The veteran accepts himself. He is what he is. Period. The veteran accepts that he did this but he did not do that. This survivor contemplates how to connect to the source, how to enjoy what is, and how to feel content. If he has not accomplished something, well, it probably is not going to get done now. Time may have run out for taking in new information. Charles Nelson said that by seventy, many people probably have lost the ability to process new data. This ability to absorb new information, however, varies with the individual and how mentally active he or she is. A veteran learns to appreciate the moment, for he realizes that each new day is a gift.

The veteran has a whole group of life experiences, events, emotions, and lessons to share with others. He is a teacher. Often older artists create their best work when they are more freed up from life's duties and expectations and have a strong sense of self. These artists can set an example for others to follow. As mental stimulation is important at all stages of life, veterans keep an active interest in some project or art. The individual profits most who learns to take advantage of all the different opportunities that each consecutive stage of life presents.

QUESTIONS TO CONSIDER

1. WHAT ARE THE LESSONS THAT YOU LEARNED FROM BEING A PARENT?

2. WHAT STAGE OF LIFE ARE YOU IN? HOW ARE YOU HANDLING IT?

3. WHAT ARE YOUR TECHNIQUES FOR STARTING OVER?

4. IS YOUR WORK SATISFYING? IN WHAT WAY?

5. DID YOU MAKE ANY CHANGES IN YOUR FIFTIES? CAREER CHANGES? LIFE CHANGES?

6. WHAT ARE YOUR PLANS FOR RETIREMENT TO REMAIN INTELLECTUALLY AND PHYSICALLY ACTIVE?

7. HAVE YOU SOUGHT OUT A NEW SOCIAL ACTIVITY LATELY? IF SO, WHAT?

Chapter VII
MENTAL STIMULATION AND ART

Art

The definition of art is an interesting one, because art can be very hard to define. Jared Diamond, in *The Third Chimpanzee,* outlines three criteria for human art: it is nonutilitarian, for aesthetic pleasure, and transmitted by learning not genes. I believe that art is not so narrowly defined but may have usefulness as well as beauty. For example, architecture is beautiful but also useful. The bridges in Portland, Oregon, spanning the Willamette River add beauty to the city's skyline, yet we still drive our cars across them.

Art is for aesthetic pleasure. We could drink water out of a tin can which is not art. If we drink water out of a beautiful, hand-made ceramic cup with graceful shape, pleasing color, and design; that is art.

Art is not transmitted by genes. In humans, the capacity for art is genetic, but it will not manifest automatically. The interest must be developed.

The arts may have begun for religious or ritual purposes, to influence nature and the supernatural. For example, the caves as Lascaux, France, where the artist drew the image of animals on the cave wall to gain power over them. The arts, however, quickly took on a life of their own and began to fill our needs for mental stimulation, spiritual uplift and emotional expression.

The arts further fulfilled our need for the expression and appreciation of beauty, and the manipulaiton of our environment. From the environment and nature came the early materials for art; such as rock, clay, plant fibers, different yarns from animal hair, and different dyes from plant material and minerals.

Unsatisfied with everyday reality, people begin to tell stories, sing songs, draw on the cave wall, decorate the teepee and beat sticks together to bring extra-natural experience and stimulation to their minds. Art is built on the expression of ideas that do not occur in nature. Many artistic motifs arise from nature but are usually modified or exaggerated in some way. Art is man-made.

Artistic creation is part of who we are as human beings. We have hands with opposable thumbs for grasping and manipulating tools and objects. Put together the learning mind seeking stimulation and the grasping hand seeking manipulation, and humans are well on the way to becoming creators and artists.

Art fills many roles. As well as being stimulating and beautiful, the arts fill specific human needs such as ownership. For example, the tribesmen or women who painted personal art on their homes did so to exhibit their individual mark. Many early designs became the property of one family, such as a Persian rug design for the family rug business.

Body ornamentation has an ancient history. Body paint, feathers, bones, earrings, nose rings, and tatoos were early artistic expressions designed to make people more beautiful, more distinctive, more attractive or more important. Body paint was used to send messages. When necessary the warrior wore body paint to signify that he was going to war. These arts of body decoration are still current today. Make-up, hair dyeing, tatooing, nose rings, jewelry, and fashionable clothing are still popular.

As well as making a visual statement, the arts serve a more serious purpose. The arts are a means to hone and sharpen our senses. For every sense, there is a corresponding art. For the ear, there is music. For the eye, there is visual art. For the hands, there is pottery and sculpture. For general body sensation, there is dancing and movement. For the mind, there is scientific creativity and inquiry: the art of thinking.

These arts develop our senses and allow for fine tuning that may not occur anywhere else. The arts develop mental skills, problem solving skills, emotional skills and motor skills. We have had art for thousands of years so it obviously plays a central role in human development and achievement.

In the past, participation in the arts was socially useful to the artist. Diamond believes that art was beneficial to the artist because it probably signalled talent, money, prestige and may therefore have helped attract a mate. Even in modern society, many people still appreciate the work of the artist.

As well as being personally beneficial, art enhances the society as well. Art contributes to the social cohesion of the society and enables members of the group to identify themselves and bond. Some of these bonding arts include drama, painting, storytelling, dance and music.

Art is emotionally satisfying for creator and observer. It expresses difficult emotions in acceptable ways. The creator expresses him or herself and passes this message to the observer to appreciate as well. Art enhances our ability to feel emotion deeply.

Art Therapy

Because it expresses emotion, art can be used as therapy for many problems that humans encounter. Ashly Prend in *Transcending Loss* gives the example of a lady whose son was killed in the Lockerbie airplane explosion. As a professional sculptor, the bereaved mother dealt with her grief by sculpting herself in all her different positions of grief. She later joined a therapy group with others who had relatives die in the same crash.

She invited them to come to her studio and pose in their position of grief at hearing the news of the loved one's death. "To see all these larger than life sculptures together is a striking experience that moves some people to tears," says Prend. Art is an accepted means to work out powerful, painful experiences as well as beautiful ones.

Since each person has individual experiences, each individual who observes art has a different reaction to it. A particular work may resonate with one observer and move that person deeply while another observer may feel nothing. That is why the artist gets such varied reactions to each piece of work that he or she creates.

Because language is a fairly recent development, it does not express all human feeling. Art can be used to express ideas and feelings that do not find successful expression in words. For instance, people involved in shattering psychological trauma can often draw pictures that describe the feelings and the terrible events that they experienced, even when the person cannot put these feelings into words. Sometimes the trauma is so shattering that the person doesn't want to put the experience into words, but can draw to vent these feelings.

Art can be used for many different psychological purposes. According to Cathy Malchiodi in *The Art Therapy Sourcebook*, art can soothe the self, release stress and tension, give enjoyment and pleasure, transcend troubled feelings, tap the intuitive, emotional, and creative powers. Art frees the personal voice which may be stifled by a person's busy life which allows no creative time. However, if that same person takes time to draw a picture, play the piano, or write in her diary; she is taking the time to connect with and express her personal, inner voice. This connection keeps the person in harmony with herself.

Art has the advantage that it can be very free-form. Malchiodi notices that in patients' drawings, ambiguous or contradictory elements can be included because art doesn't have the same rigid rules about structure and organization as everyday language normally does. However, language can also be free-form and expressive in poetry and the more creative areas of language. As well as drawing for expression, a person can write in a diary for self-expression and therapeutic purposes.

Art therapy is especially beneficial, because in the world of psychology, it is one of the few areas where the patient can actually perform an action that will produce potentially pleasing and tangible results. The concept of creating something real and visible is an extra reward in itself.

Malchiodi reminds us that "Through art making one can also experiment with new ideas, new ways of expression, and new ways of seeing. Finding joy, playing, creating, and communicating in a meaningful way are necessary for psychological, physical, and spiritual health. Making art provides these experiences."

Four areas are especially strong influences on the arts: mental stimulation, language, sex, and aggression. These four areas will be covered in the following pages.

Art helps in situations of mental deprivation to stimulate the brain.

The arts provide a variety of services for mankind, especially in situations where the person needs extra stimulation.

- Art provides mental stimulation. There is an art to stimulate every human sense. Many arts, like social dance, simultaneously stimulate many senses.

- Art provides an accepted means of expression for ideas and feelings that are unable to be expressed any other way. Possibly, a means to express emotions that are not able to be spoken with any clarity.

- Art provides short-term or long-term goals for a person who is having difficult making himself move forward in his daily life.

- Learning an art provides mental stimulation and satisfaction to the person who may be low on self-esteem and needs to generate some feelings of self-worth.

- Many arts, like social dancing, playing basketball, or singing in a choir, are a good way to be around people and form friendships.

- Art promotes the development of perceptual thinking for "the most effective training of perceptual thinking can be found in the art studio," says Arnheim in *Visual Thinking*.

- Art sets the brain to work on constructive thinking, rather than dwelling on less pleasant thoughts. It is a positive mental distraction.

- As a means to create novelty, art stimulation keeps the mind busy and helps to prevent dementia, depression, and Altzheimer's which may all be due in part to reduced stimulation.

- Some arts, like pottery, painting, and sculpting, result in a physical, tangible creation that may be enjoyed and admired for a long time. The creation stands as a visible symbol of the artists self expression.

Through all the different aspects of social and sensory deprivation, the arts can play a major role in keeping the human in balance.

Language as the Basis for Representation

Language is the first symbol system that makes way for all the other symbolic systems that follow such as art and mathematics. It lets us hear a sound or see a written letter as the representation for a real thing. This basis of symbolic representation paves the way for artistic expression, since art also makes use of symbolic systems. The use of language comes in many different forms.

• *Storytelling*

One of the first uses of symbolism is storytelling which has held a special place in human culture since ancient times when the history of society was passed down orally. The tribal elders, who were the historians and sages of their people, were valued for their skill in remembering and reciting long oral traditions such as epic poems or the geneology of the tribe. The tribe gathered around the campfire and the elders began to tell various important events that had taken place, about the myth of creation or warriors in heroic battles. Thus, the elder in the tribe was a repository of vital information, much like a modern encyclopedia.

With more accomplished speech plus a longer lifespan, Cro-Magnon gave prominence to the elders and story telling. Jared Diamond in *Guns, Germs and Steel*, describes a storyteller in a New Guinea village who knew where to find plants that could be eaten in an emergency, such as a drought. When the drought came, this elder was the only person who knew how to survive. "One such person in a preliterate society can thus spell the difference between death and survival for the whole society," says Diamond. Thus, longevity, storytelling and the information held within these stories had a definite evolutionary advantage.

Many religions have great storytelling traditions to pass on lessons of morality, creation, and religious practices. Storytelling, which was often a great social event, allowed societies to explain the beginning of the universe and all its mysteries. Storytelling became ritualistic for special occasions, such as a religious ceremony or a modern day church service.

Storytelling, like writing in a diary, is therapeutic to the health. "A recent study revealed that patients given the opportunity to tell their stories before surgery recovered more quickly. Stories are regularly used in health care today, especially in gerontology and psychotherapy," says Caren Neile in an article on "Storytelling" in *The Toastmaster*.

Scholars think of humans as storytelling animals because the human brain appears to be hard-wired with the genetic disposition to both tell and retain information better when it is presented through narrative, says Neile. There is no culture on earth that does not have some stories. One example is the American Indians, with a strong storytelling history, the word was sacred and was used to influence the spirit world and raise humans to a higher level. "The poem, the chant, the legend of migration, and the origin myth were magical utterances in the strictest sense of the term," says Leroy Appleton in *American Indian Design and Decoration.* The telling of myths, legends, and children's stories were rarely for amusement because these stories were an integral part of tribal life. In many cases they were regarded as a sacred inheritance.

Storytelling occurs in a variety of forms in modern society as when a person introduces himself to another, when the lawyer sums up the evidence for the jury in the courtroom, and when the boss tells jokes at the office to relax the workers. Creative storytelling remains a vital part of society though its form has mutated to include novels, films and television.

•*Public Speaking*

Public speaking is different from storytelling in that it is usually for a more practical purpose and not solely for enjoyment. It is usually to incite the public to some action. The Greeks and the Romans both had strong traditions of public speaking where important citizens tried to turn public opinion around or to stir the masses to some specific action, such as going to war or plotting against the govenment.

We carry on this public speaking tradition by means of television, lectures and rallies. In the United

States today, in our political elections, two presidential candidates square off for public debate so that the voters can see what ability they have as speaker and thinker. Both our legal and political systems are based on public speaking: the first is based on the ability of the lawyers to debate in court and win over the opinion of the jury, while the second seeks to win public support for reelection. Public speaking remains important in modern America.

Drama and Acting

When the first Cro-Magnon returned to the cave and acted out the adventues of the hunt, he mesmerized his audience with his voice, gestures, actions, and delivery. Soon, instead of a one-man act, he invited his friends to represent the bison he was hunting. Thus was drama born. Naturally, drama has close ties to storytelling. Early drama often had a supernatural, religious element. For instance, the group would act out the drama to scare away an evil spirit.

Drama is a time-honored way of presenting larger-than-life situations to express an idea vital to the community. For instance, in *Inherit the Wind,* a dramatization by Jerome Lawrence and Robert E. Lee of the famous "monkey trials," where the idea of evolution versus creationism is debated. Drama promotes peaceful, serious debate.

Theater is still alive and well today and is often considered the training ground for actors and producers who may then migrate to TV or the movies. In the movies, an actor can redo the scene ten times. In live theater, there is one chance to build a rapport with the audience. Thus, theater has an immediacy that TV lacks. Theater explores problems of human existence, psychological and social interactions, the fears of the society, and spiritual and emotional events of the individual or the community.

Jerry Pickering, in his book entitled *Theater,* states that "the dramatic experience can be defined as a discovery by an audience of some profound truth about humanity's existence. It is a discovery of truth through theatrical action rather than scientific inquiry, history, or philosophical thinking."

Reading and Writing

Reading and writing have added immensely to creatively and stimulation. Individuals gain knowledge both by writing themselves or by reading what others have written. Over the centuries, humans have demonstrated a great respect for the written word.

Writing was the process whereby humans finally freed themselves of the necessity to remember data by oral tradition. The earliest uses of writing found in the Near East were for business transactions. Sumerian is thought to be the first writing in 3100 BC. It was called cuneiform, a wedge-shaped script made with chisels in wet clay, and it developed from pictographs like the form of writing used by the ancient Egyptians. Chinese writing started out as pictographs but was modified somewhat to make for simpler and more beautiful writing. In the Near East and Europe came the idea of an alphabet with individual letters. Most modern European languages use an alphabet while many Asian languages have retained syllabic characters, such as Chinese.

In modern society, people are totally dependent on writing for recording births, deaths, business deals, legal agreements, stating laws, electing officials, and passing information. Society could not operate without the written word, either on the internet or on the page.

With the acceptance of writing, the village storyteller went out of business. Memorizing the genealogy of the society disappeared when it became much easier to write the information in book form. With the onset of the computer, the book may eventually vanish in the same way as the storyteller.

At present, we are still in the written society. With writing comes the necessity to read, the ability to understand the written symbols and interpret them into meaningful ideas. In early times, the general populace didn't read or write; these skills were left to the wealthy and to experts called scribes who wrote and read messages for hire. Fortunately, with public education, everyone in the US has the chance to learn to read and write.

In the computer age, average citizens are more likely to desk-top publish themselves. Writers can post works on the internet for others to read without even actually being published in book form. Writing remains a useful and necessary skill. The ability to record thinking and information has added greatly to our ability to learn and has enhanced our ability to remember.

•Sex Inspires Art

As sex is one of the elements that drives our lives and our arts, it merits discussion. Just as writing is one of our basic symbol systems, so sex is one of our most basic emotional, physical drives. Sex plays a big role in the survival of the species and therefore in its creativity. Matt Ridley, in his book *The Red Queen*, states that sex is at the foundation of what it is to be human and the driving force for human evolution. Any human characteristic that enhanced reproduction of the species had an advantage over time.

Taking the animal kingdom as a whole, human sexual habits are unusual. The first unusual trait, says Diamond in *The Third Chimpanzee*, is that humans usually have sex in private for enjoyment, rather than mainly in public and only when the female is able to conceive. Nobody really know the reason for this, but one possible explanation is that the female, being available at all times and not visibly in heat, holds the attention and interest of the male in order to keep the family unit together for an extended period of time to raise the young.

Throughout the animal kingdom, there are basically two types of mate selection for males. One where the male competes with other males to win the female, and one where the male woos the female. Both techniques select for the best males genetically, says Ridley, but the first technique selects for male bruisers and the second for male dandies. For example, the bull elephant seal and the red deer stag are huge and dangerous, while peacocks and nightingales compete aesthetically. For humans, there seems to be a choice of either way to win the female. Historically, some human males fought other males to show how strong they were, while other human males sought to win the female by flowers, candy, and music. The male may use the arts to woo the female. Once again, the human proves to be an imaginative and flexible animal.

As expected, human mate selection is a serious matter, especially for the female. The human female must find a mate that will stay with her and help her care for and teach the young for a long period of time. As a result, human females are quite selective when they go looking for a mate. On the other hand, the human male is less selective, says Diamond. The only characteristic where the male is more selective than the female turns out to be the concept of physical attractiveness. But, contrary to common thought, the concept of physical attractiveness turns out to be quite important as an overall indicator of physical health.

People who are healthier have more symmetrical features and formation. Many diseases cause impairments that are visible to those of the opposite sex who are looking for the best genes. It is safe to conclude that the most attractive, most symmetically formed people are usually the healthiest and the most likely to have good genetic stock. Throughout history, physical attractiveness has been an indication of whether or not the individual hosted parasites, since many parasites, such as ringworm and fleas, leave visible marks. Naturally, the individual looks for a mate who is not infested with parasites.

However, there is the chance of attractiveness being overdone. Sometimes humans, either male or female, who have extremely exaggerated traits that are normally considered attractive may not genetically be the best choice for a mate.

"Selection of sex partners is another important piece of what defines humanity. It's as basic to our rise from chimpanzee status as is our remodeled pelvis. We'll see that much of what we think of as human racial variation may have risen as a by-product of the beauty standards by which we pick our bedmates." says Diamond.

Through the ages, before the advent of large standing armies and large countries, sex was a main reasons for starting wars, says Diamond. Famous stories like Helen of Troy and the war that ensued are actually realistic. Sex has also been one of the main causes of crimes committed by social misfits. Sex is obviously an extremely important element in the shaping of the human, the human arts, the human family and human society. Love and sex test our ability to successfully get along with our fellow humans.

Since the human selection of sexual partners is based on the idea of symmetry and beauty, this same love of symmetrical beauty, says, Ridley, is extrapolated to the world as a whole. Objects that are symmetrical and beautiful are, in the human mind, considered artistic and attractive. Our methods of mate seletion help us create and appreciate symmetry in life and in art. In addition, the drive to find a mate provides very strong feelings for humans so these powerful emotions have, through the ages, often found their expression in magnificent art works.

•Aggression Inspires Art

An interesting experience was reported by Jane Goodall, a scientist who has studied chimpanzees all her life. At first, she wondered why the chimpanzees she studied in the wild were such mild, pleasant beings and why humans were so aggressive. She was puzzled about the difference in behavior. Then one day, the troop of chimpanzees that she was studying went to the neighboring troop and created havoc, killing most of the other troop. Then she understood. Violence is just part of chimpanzee life and behavior.

Aggression and violence are present to some degree in all human and chimpanzee societies and are central to the human condition and human expression. As such, much of art and music was designed to be used in battle to invigorate the army, unite the fighters, and strike terror into the hearts of the enemy. Hence, the introduction of horns, drums, bagpipes, banners, shield art, coat of arms, national flags, and military uniforms. Aggression is a likely impetus behind instrumental band music.

The warrior's war paint makes him more frightening and less human thereby demonstrating how art enhances aggression. The uniform created for soldiers going into war identified them as a group that was all united for a single purpose. The medals given for valor on the field are beautiful and impressive. Art helps to show importance and rank in the military.

As humans have become more confined in civilization rather than roaming on the African savannah, citizens often have more difficulty expressing their aggression. To this end, both the arts and sports are beneficial to the person who needs to vent emotionally.

A large part of the creativity of the human race has been devoted to making a bigger and better catapult to strike the enemy. Often our creativity in weaponry has led the way to inventions that add to the society in peace time. For instance, the rockets that were originally designed to deliver war heads to the enemy have now evolved to carry humans to outer space.

Art and the Computer

Graphic arts are artistic expression combined with the written word. Computer art, especially in the field of graphic arts for magazines, newspapers, brochures, advertising and other commercial art uses, has changed the field dramatically. Photos can now be scanned into the computer or entered into the computer by means of a digital camera to make the photograph part of the graphic presentation. These photos can be redesigned at will. Color printers can then print out the final copy immediately without all the old hands-on layout, set-up, and expensive printing. These processes have revolutionized the world of printing.

The computer has many wonderful uses but also some drawbacks. Continual computer use affects people mentally and physically since sitting in front of the computer monitor may be harmful to the health. Watching the monitor screen for long periods of time is hard on the eyes even with eye protection. Studies have shown that when some people sit in front of a computer for too long, they not only get physical problems like back and neck strain, possible carpal tunnel injuries in the hands, but also possible mental symptoms like irritability. In addition, sitting in front of screens can cause lack of exercise and obesity. Computers are a necessary component of modern life but need to be used intelligently.

High tech is changing the arts. The field of music

now has synthesizers that can produce the sound of any musical instrument all in one place without orchestra or conductor; yet, people still attend concerts with live musicians. It seems that the onslaught of high tech in music has not so far lessened the appeal of traditional music.

Howver, electronic keyboards have become very popular, cutting heavily into the sales of traditional pianos. The electronic keyboard is much lighter and more mobile for bands that travel a lot. Yet, the traditional piano remains.

Though art has gone high tech, it still requires individual artistic input. High tech has opened up new worlds for art; one dramatic example is in the movie industry, where once primitive special effects now look absolutely real. The sky is the limit. Yet, the ability to create drawings and artistic forms is one of our oldest arts and will remain a valued skill.

QUESTIONS TO CONSIDER

1. HOW DO YOU DEFINE ART?

2. HAVE YOU EVER USED ART FOR THERAPEUTIC PURPOSES? IN WHAT WAY?

3. IN WHAT WAYS DO YOU CREATIVELY USE LANGUAGE?

4. DO SEX OR AGGRESSION PLAY A ROLE IN YOUR ARTISTIC EXPRESSION? IF SO, HOW?

5. WHAT ROLE WILL COMPUTER PLAY IN THE FUTURE OF ART AND SELF EXPRESSION?

Chapter VIII

THE POWER OF MUSIC AND OTHER ARTS

I have come to believe that music is the art that effects us most powerfully and thus deserves a featured place of its own. Early experience with music and its pleasant associations are the reason that music is primary. Music is one of our first exposures, for our introduction to sound and rhythm starts even before birth. When the baby is in utero, he hears the rhythm of the mother's heartbeat and the sound of her voice as she sings or speaks his language. Since sound travels well in water, it is obvious that the baby is hearing, whereas touch, taste, smell and sight are still a ways down the road. Thus the unborn baby and the newborn baby both associate music, especially music that has about the same rhythm as a heart beat, with comfort and security. Dr. Lee Salk, says Shelley Katsh in *Music Within You*, discovered that newborns actually do better in preschools where a recording of a human heart-beat is being played continuously.

A singer who performed at weddings during her pregnancy had her baby. She noticed that her newborn baby was humming as she left the hospital after the baby's birth. The baby had heard a lot of music prior to being born and already knew how to express herself in music.

Because music is central to human expression, it has a long history. The Cro-Magnon had musical instruments which included the flute and the rattle over 40,000 years ago. Some believe that music started even earlier. Josie Glausiusz in "The Genetic Mystery of Music' in *Discover Magazine*, believes that music started sometime between 43,000 and 82,000 years ago when a Neanderthal living in a cave in what is now Slovenia fashioned a flute from the femur of a bear. Simple instruments such as rattles and drums probably preceded it, and singing probably began even earlier, perhaps as long as 250,000 years ago.

Joan Goldsmith in *How Can We Keep From Singing,* tells of two French explorers, Reynikoff and Dauvois, who explored Neanderthal and Cro-Magnon caves in France. As they explored these caves, they sang and discovered that the caves adorned with the most art had the best acoustics; thus suggesting the interesting possibility that the caverns might have been used for multimedia presentations in caveman days.

It seems that the potential for music and enjoyment of it is an innate characteristic of humans. Glausiusz describes the music experimentation performed on young children by Sandra Trehub at the University of Toronto. In the study, a machine played a series of notes and periodically played a note that did not fit in. The young children listening to the music picked up on the incorrect note immediately. "I'm convinced that there's a biological basis for the babies' abilities," says Trehub.

However, music, like many other human skills, needs early encouragement to develop fully; even toddlers can successfully benefit from music lessons. Children like to hear music sung to them at an early age, especially when it is sung to them by their parents. The children then begin to mimic the singing of their parents and quickly learn to sing themselves. A child of two can sing a specific melody.

Some believe that music has a timeline where it can best be entered and past that date, it is difficult or impossible to master. Music, says Klawans in *Defending the Cavewoman*, is an acquired skill which must be started before the age of 13 to be mastered successfully.

Music can affect mood. Music can transform a bad mood into a more pleasant one. As stated before, the heart beat relaxes the young child and this relaxation response to music continues into adulthood. Music soothes the spirit. Listening to music makes us forget our problems. It is the one rather passive activity that still has a beneficial effect on the brain as opposed to TV and other passive pursuits which do not.

Music has the ability to soothe pain. Since it stimulates the pleasure centers, it can remove us to a place of pleasure and distract us from the pain that we feel. For instance, many people can dance for long hours at a time but do not realize that their feet hurt because they are enjoying the act of dancing to music so thoroughly. Music can distract a patient who is receiving minor surgery or dentistry. The patient can concentrate on the music and rise above the anxiety and discomfort of the procedure.

Cognitive and emotional skills are both required for music: cognitive skills to create music and learn to play it, and emotional skills to make it beautiful. Those who interact with music have more emotional development because of the musical contact.

Music stimulates mental abilities. The music of Mozart is especially beneficial to young listeners with rapidly learning brains. Thus the beneficial effects of music are sometimes called the "Mozart Effect." A possible explanation of the Mozart Effect may be due to beat. The average heartbeat is 72-80 beats per minute which coincides with the average tempo of Western (European) music, according to Shelley Katsh in *The Music Within You*.

Rock music or other types of more strident music are not as beneficial as Mozart perhaps because the tempo is different.

Music is beneficial to cognitive development. Don Campbell in his book called *The Mozart Effect*, states that music stimulates brain growth, enhances motor development, improves reading, writing, math, and other academic skills, promotes self-identity, and enhances spatial perception and intelligence temporarily. Many mathematicians and scientists are also musicians.

Music stimulates the pleasure centers of the brain and adds to our ability to experience joy. Watch the looks on the faces of any instrumentalist, singer, or dancer who is deep into the performance of music. It is almost like they are on a different plane of existence and feeling nothing but joy. When a musician is involved with music, it prevents the cognitive thought center from thinking about everyday problems. Perhaps the emotional system may be able to take over the conscious brain during the experience of pleasure as well as during a crisis.

Both vocal and instrumental music can affect us deeply. It reaches the psyche and the soul. Music sends chills up and down the spine, especially for the performer in concert who is right in the center of the musical event while it is happening with real surround sound.

Music helps promote mate selection. Darwin thought that early humans were unable to express their love with words, so they "endeavored to charm each other with musical notes and rhythm," as birds do, says Glausiusz. Hence the Italian tradition of serenading a prospective mate where the male lover stands beneath the window singing to his intended.

Another study supporting the relationship between music and mate selection was conducted by Geoffrey Miller, an evolutionary psychologist at the University of New Mexico. He noticed in all genres of music, men produce about 10 times as much as women and their output peaks at around 30—near the peak reproductive years, writes Glausiusz.

Team work and human bonding occurs in music just as in sports. A band, choir, or orchestra is many people working together for the united effort and common good. In an orchestra, everyone is coordinated by means of counting and by means of the conductor who holds the group together. Each player has a part that contributes to the whole, the final production, that is greater than the sum of its parts.

Music is a social event. Music can be played solo, but ultimately it takes other people, whether as audience or participants, to really make it a worthwhile experience. Of course, playing with music groups is immediately social.

Music promotes social contact; it proves beneficial to the community as an outlet for tension. Music helps people get along with each other. Hajime Fukui at the Nara University of Education Japan believes that music alleviates sexual tension by lowering men's testosterone levels. He believes that music was used in early societies to reduce sexual tension and to help the society function peacefully together, writes Glausiusz. A good example of this cooperation is folk dances and songs that channel human behavior into fixed, musical expression for special occasions, such as weddings.

People are attracted by music. If someone hears beautiful music, he will want to stop and listen. Music brings joy to other people. People who play must realize that their performance allows those who don't play to hear music. A musical performer is the conduit between the composer and the audience.

People who create music get their joy from the act of creation. People who perform music get satisfaction by bringing the joy of music to others. Musicians would not enjoy it half so much if there were no one to listen to their performance, for the act of performing makes the player rise to his highest skill level. People who enjoy listening to music get their musical experience from hearing and appreciating the production of music. All three aspects are part of the whole.

When we play a musical instrument, we ultimately get more out of it than when we simply listen to music. Playing makes the musician submerge himself deeper and requires skills and brain development over a period of time. Listening to music is great, but performance challenges our brain more intensely.

To control all the variables of music takes real focus and repetition. It requires time for it to happen for music is a long-term project that takes hours of practice and years of study to master. Learning music teaches the student not to expect immediate gratification.

Unfortunately, many people can't stick it out and never get to the stage where they can really enjoy the instrument. Many people choose an instrument, play for six months or less if they are lucky, then give up because the instrument required more time and patience than they could give.

Music requires total concentration which is advantageous if the musician has troubles. The positive experience of playing can drowned out any other mental thoughts. Thus, music becomes a positive experience and a buffer against the negative aspects of life.

Music aids in memory. There are many rules to follow in music and the player has to remember all the rules in order to produce music that others can enjoy or music to play with others. In addition, many soloist instrumentalists or vocalists memorize large works so that they can put more emotion into their performance. Once the music is memorized, the artist is free to add the expression and emotion without worrying about the details of reading the notes and turning the pages. Memorizing the work makes the performer more free to bond with the audience and look at them without being distracted by notation details.

The successful student learns to take charge of what he learns. The student may tell the private teacher that his preferences are for a certain kind of music and that he does not want to learn any other. Or, he may just spend a lot of personal time playing the music that he likes. A student has to let the teacher know what he is willing to learn or learn it on his own.

Piano as an Example

As an example of learning a common instrument, the physical requirements of piano are demanding. Piano takes a lot of manual dexterity. The student must learn to play one pattern with the left hand (the percussion) and another with the right (usually the melody.) Both hands have to learn to move separately. One hand may be going down the keyboard while the other is going up, or one hand may be playing one rhythm with the other hand playing a different rhythm.

Each finger must learn to move separately. The weaker fingers like the fourth finger and the little finger learn to move individually. When each hand is doing something different, the piano player memorizes one hand so that it will be automatic in order to concentrate on the other. Piano strengthens the fingers like few other activities. The fingers learn to move quickly over the keys in different, ever changing patterns.

Piano also teaches eye-hand coordination. The piano player sees the notes on the page and translates them into hand movements. This habit takes several years to master. It takes time before the hands can find the notes by touch. This is much the same skill that is gained by the hands on a computer keyboard.

Reading music includes seeing changes in notes and note groups, associating pitch with rising and falling note patterns, and rhythmic notation as well as dynamic marking such as fast, slow, loud, and soft. Rhythm may include pulses in two, three, and four beats or combinations of these pulses to produce such complex rhythms such as five, seven, and nine.

The music student learns to sight read which is a very complex skill. Sight reading is when the student sits down to a piece of music he has never seen before and plays it with some degree of credibility. If the student has not practiced the assigned music; come lesson time, the student has to be able to sightread well enough to convince the teacher that she has at least spent some time playing that particular piece.

Reading music includes learning which notes go together, what are the intervals between notes, and which blocks of notes operate as one unit, as one might recognize a word. These skills have to register quickly and translate into action in the course of playing. In truth, music and language may use some of the same areas of the brain, reports Burkhard Maess and associates from Germany, because both music and language are rule-based notation systems.

Choral Music

Choral music, often coupled with orchestra, makes a moving, powerful statement; it combines our need to speak words and our love of melody and harmony. Singing, especially in groups, has a special appeal for humanity. Joan Goldsmith states that 20 million American (10.4 % of us) perform in choral groups, according to the National Endowment for the Arts.

In Eugene, Oregon, May, 2001, a wonderful example of the social power of music took place. A local man was dying of cancer who had been previously active within the musical arts, both in choirs and in supporting the symphony orchestra. When the Eugene Symphony almost went bankrupt, he stepped in and prevented it. When he knew that he was dying, he wanted to leave a free performance of Brahm's "Requiem," his favorite piece of music, for the community of Eugene to enjoy.

He lined up Marin Alsop, a well-known visiting conductor, to lead the Eugene Symphony. He asked 130 willing singers from the community to volunteer for the choir. He planned to attend but, unfortunately, he died before the performance so the work became his own requiem. It was a powerful tribute to his love for music. The production, which cost over $75,000 dollars, was paid for out of his own pocket, and was enormously moving both to the participants and to the audience. It was an unforgettable moment. Of course, Brahm's "Requiem" is a tremendously powerful piece of music and memorable in its own right.

Choral groups combine the powerful human social need with the love of song. When choral groups sing harmony together, it takes very close listening and makes the group work very closely and intently together. Most people belong to choirs just for the sheer spiritual uplift and comraderie a choir can provide. Choral music gets right down to the human soul. Most amateur choirs have a good time because the people assemble with the sole idea of enjoying themselves. A choral experience gives people a break from the stresses of everyday existence serves as a mental vacation, and creates spiritual fulfillment.

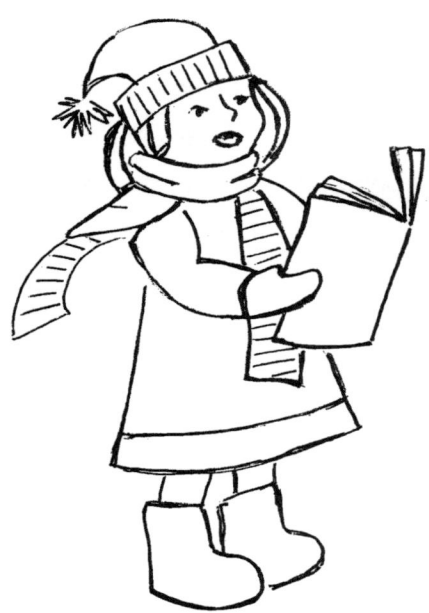

Painting and Drawing as Mental Stimulation

Humans gain the ability to understand representation at an early age. Any normal one-and a-half to two-year old child can tell that a stick figure represents mommy and daddy, though the child does not yet have the ability to draw the stick figure. From our ability to understand representation comes the desire to create art, for art is the use of skill and imagination to create representations.

The history of the visual arts is an ancient one. In European history, some of the art in caves in France dates back to around 40,000 years ago with the arrival of Cro-Magnon. One of the most famous of these sites is the cave at Lascaux, France where cave murals depict such animals as bison, elk, deer, and bear. The drawings at Lascaux gave the Cro-Magnons power over the animals that they hunted in order to succeed better at the hunt. This art was given great value and was appreciated by the whole society.

The role of present day art is very different. In modern times, the artist is often isolated. Within large cities, it becomes progressively harder for an artist to even make his creation visible to the whole community let alone be appreciated. The modern artist must be a successful entrepreneur and work hard to get his product before the viewing public.

The artist must be an innovator and be able to

turn nothing into something. The artist takes the bare canvas and creates a beautiful painting, takes the lump of clay and makes a beautiful ceramic, takes the pile of wood and creates a home.

Light is important to the artist. Since we live on a planet warmed by the sun, we are naturally attracted to and affected by light. Light affects our mood and our energy levels. Light allows us to see color. These colors in turn affect the way that we feel about our environment. Warm colors, such as red, tend to make us feel active, while cool colors, such as blue, tend to make us more calm. Green seems to be a neutral color in the middle. We are affected by the color of the walls in our home and the color of clothing that we wear.

The artist uses many elements such as distance, size difference, color difference, parallel and convergent lines, perspective, light and dark, shadow, and reflection. Dealing with so many variables causes the artist to develop a keen eye. The workings of the eye of the artist are more complex than most imagine. The artistic processes of the eye further include exploration, selection of subject, grasping of the essentials that make that subject, simplification, abstraction, analysis and synthesis. Furthermore, completion, correction, comparison, problem solving, combining, separating, and putting in context are all performed by the eye, says Rudolph Arnheim in *Visual Thinking*. All these skills are essential to art and are sharpened by the artist.

The artist has to mentally see what he wants to create. Art requires the use of the imagination, says Daniel Druback in *The Brain Explained*. Imagination works like a laboratory for rehearsing actions, creation, and problem solving. As a result, when the artist uses her imagination, she is practicing and enhancing the human ability to solve visual problems. The use of the eyes in art trains the artist to better notice visual detail and detect problems. Art is a productive skill builder.

The artist uses depth perception, the skill that developed for swinging through the trees, for perspective. Perspective is the ability to show the relationship between items that are near and far. The cave drawings at Lascaux show perspective, for the animals in the distance are smaller; those in front are larger. In addition, those in front cover up those in the back.

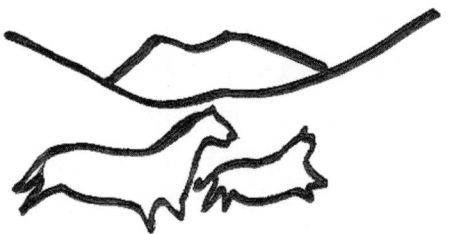

Drawing and painting teach hand-eye coordination. Contrary to the traditional expectation, the artist does not need to be able to draw a straight line, but the artist does need a steady hand.

Traps for the Artist

There are many traps to ensnare the artist. One trap is the necessity for long-term vision. David Bayles in *Art and Fear*, speaks of artists who dream of having their own one man show. When they get this opportunity, they never create another thing. The artists had no vision what to do after they completed the one man show, the short-term goal. They had no plans for the future.

Bayles regrets that artists often quit too soon. The job of the artist, according to Bayles, is to keep working to get through the periods of learning, make the necessary mistakes, and finally reach his own voice. In this quest, life experience is an asset to the artist. Often the artist creates some of his best work when he is older and has been through more of life's complications and ordeals which add depth to his work. As the artist matures, so does emotional understanding which shows more profoundly in later works. Coming into one's own as an artist requires time as well as application.

Being an artist requires constant application. If the artist takes a break, there is always the fear that his skill will disappear. Matter of fact, after a long break, some of the skill has disappeared so it takes a while to get back into the act of creation and doing that particular art form. Art, like all skills, diminishes with lack of use.

It is in the act of doing that art is created. Bayles

tells of a professor of art who told his students that he would divide the class in half. One half would be graded on volume of art produced while the other half would be graded on producing one fine piece. At the end of the class, it was the quantity side which also produced the finest pieces. More effort increases the chance of success. Those who sit around trying to visualize or create the one perfect piece never succeed. The artist who generates new ideas on a steady basis and has the craft and perseverence to carry the work to completion will succeed. Therefore, the two basic ingredients to the successful art work are inspiration plus steady application.

For the artist, there is always the fear that creativity and talent have dried up. "Talent, if it is anything, is a gift, and nothing of the artist's own making," says Bayles. "Talent is a snare and a delusion. In the end, the practical questions about talent come down to these: Who cares? Who would know? and What difference would it make? And the practical answers are: Nobody, Nobody, and None." Most success in the arts is due to repetition and practice, which give the artist the ability to begin the work, get through the difficult spots, see it through to completion.

Unfortunately, art is a field where teaching brings more income than doing. Many artists teach in order to survive. Most art professors at universities have teaching demands that deprive them of the time and energy to practice their chosen vocation.

Society does not make it easy for the artist to remain an artist. There are few jobs or ways for the beginning artist to find income. Most artists decide that they can't do art to earn a living. This is a terrible waste for society, the arts, and the artist. "If ninety-eight percent of our medical students were no longer practicing medicine five years after graduation, there would be a Senate investigation, yet that proportion of art majors are routinely consigned to an early professional death, " says Bayles. The artist has to fight to remain in the field.

The artistic persona requires a bit of fortitude, for the artist cannot be unduly swayed by public reaction. An observer who compliments on one day will turn around and criticize on another day. As a result, the artist quickly learns that artistic opinion is not carved in stone. In the end, the artist pleases herself for the compliment or criticism often says more about the state of mind of the observer than the merit of the work.

Many people like to criticize and point out errors or aspects of the artwork that they would change. Sometimes this is very helpful, such as an architect giving helpful advice on how to paint the angles of the house in the picture. Yet other times, the critic does not have useful information or advice and is just being negative. The artist quickly learns to spot the difference between the two.

Sometimes the artist gets caught up in a persona that the public creates for her. The public likes to believe that there is something superhuman and mysterious about the artist, which can work to the advantage of the artist in sales and general mystique. Many artists with good stage presence and a good business sense, revel in this elevated, exaggerated role.

Characteristics of the Visual Artist

Who does art and what characteristics define the artist? These traits were given in reference to the visual artist; however, many apply to artist in other fields as well. Howard Gardner in *The Arts and Human Development* lists some of the characteristics that many artists share. Some are quite surprising.

- The lack of a father is common feature for artists, who not infrequently have lost one or even both parents at an early age.

- The artist often has a heightened consciousness of self and a sense of mission with regard to the world.

- The artist often has a particular degree of self-confidence.

- Many artist have unusual religious backgrounds.

- The childhood home of the artist includes an assortment of interesting, creative personalities.

- Often a malady or some pivotal event in childhood seems to have been formative for artists. This situation creates deep emotions that the artist seeks to express by way of his or her art.

- The setting of the early years plays an important part. Often there are beautiful landscapes, frequent music, and other activities that would encourage the arts.

- Sometimes an artist divides himself into two entities: the normal self and the creative self.

- Many artists have had heated conflict with a parent, usually the father.

- The artist requires a range of experiences and feeling to express his art. A varied background is vital to the development of the artist.

- The artist usually has a heightened awareness of shape and color.

- The artist slowly evolves a characteristic way of interpreting experience so that a dominant personal style begins to emerge.

- Often an artist has a reversal as going from rich to poor.

It is conceivable that a visual artist has a heightened sense of shape and color. Other characteristics such as argumentation with a father, having no father, might cause a person to need extra self-expression. Perhaps the difference between the artist and the non-artist is somewhat a question of need. With bad times, the artist looks to art for expression while the non-artist may have other avenues to express himself.

The artist needs the stimulation of bright colors and aesthetically pleasing items in the environment. For this reason, artists often decorate their homes with exotic artwork or wear bright colors which may seem unusual to other people. For an artist who is used to having visual stimulation, bare, ivory colored walls is not a home. White walls are for institutions and hospitals. White walls are visual deprivation and torture for the artist.

Betty Edwards in *Drawing on the Right Side of the Brain* believes that visual art is easily accessible to everyone. For her, drawing simply includes the ability to notice and define edges, observe light and shadow, create space and contour, notice relationships in size and arrangement, and observe the gestalt or how the parts fit into the whole. With these skills, anyone can draw.

By combining these elements together, the artist has the opportunity to make a statement larger than life. If the artist wants to emphasize some attribute more than another and distort reality to this end, he has this opportunity. Since the artist has the chance to bend reality to his or her will, he or she learns to take control of the environment.

Many fields take years before the person is ready to start. However, art is one field where the student can learn by trial and error and imitation. The art student can learn by doing. The adventurous student can pick an art, get advice from a successful artist or read a book that explains the process, get the supplies, and see what develops. If the art can be done without a teacher, fine. If help and demonstrations are needed, then he seeks a talented teacher who is not too invasive.

Many times the beginning artist can work on her own and just ask advice occasionally of another artist when a specific problem arises. Most artists like to share information with beginners about how to solve various problems. By joining an art guild, the art student can find artists who will answer questions, have some social contact, and learn a lot just by watching and asking questions about the art that other artists bring to the group. Everyone starts some place and the beginner cannot be shy. Art is in the doing of it.

Visual arts promote the well-being of the brain. According to Semir Zeki in *The Scientific American Book of the Brain,* visual stimulation causes an increased blood flow to the visual cortex which causes better health in that area. Therefore, stimulation of the different senses by different art forms is good for the brain and, as a result, good for a person's overall health.

The History of the Building Arts.

Around the seventh millennium BC, people living in the Fertile Crescent, the area between the Euphrates and Tigris Rivers in the Middle East, had gained the skills of agriculture, crafts, and trade and were settled in one place, thus began the rise of cities. As the city began so did the art of construction. Permanent homes, shrines, temples, gardens, and palaces were added to the experience of what it is to be human. An example is Jericho, which is considered the oldest city, that was built around 8000 BC. Most of the houses in Jericho were made of mud bricks, according to Jonathan Glancey in *The Story of Architecture.*

Houses, as one of our most central structures, play many different roles in our lives. They protect us from the elements, give us privacy, promote the family unit, and give us areas to store our belongings, necessities, and crafts. Homes give us an area to sleep that is protected from wandering wild animals, marauding humans, and bad weather. In addition, homes were the first places of business. Later on, homes became declarations of wealth and prestige.

From the first simple homes, construction advanced quickly. Historically, the first real examples of architecture were temples, the first of which was the Ziggurat, a sort of step pyramid. This was probably the model for the Tower of Babel in the Bible.

Fine examples of architecture were discovered in Babylon, Yemen, Persia, Iran, Iraq, Egypt, and Africa. For the Western World, architecture was felt to hit its stride with the rise of Classical Greece. In Golden Age of Greece, two buildings stand out: the Acropolis built around 800 BC and the Parthenon around 500 BC. The buildings of Greece were the first examples of construction made for utility, beauty, and enjoyment. Many of these Greek buildings were very popular with the people, and the Greeks spent much of their lives under the columns of these wonderful buildings.

Greek architecture went world-wide. Many countries even today have buildings that are built to resemble the Greek style, especially government buildings that need to be impressive. Probably one of the most useful and popular public structures borrowed from the Greeks is the theater/stadium. These stadiums are often build into the hillside with rows of seats in a semi-circular arrangement. As a local example, just about every high school in the United States has some type of stadium for pep rallies and other school events.

The popular Greek building tradition was furthered and improved by the Romans around 100 AD. The Romans excelled in building fine structures such as the Coloseum in Rome where many public spectacles were held. We owe much of our present day knowledge about the building arts to the early works of both the Greeks and the Romans.

The Romans invented concrete, made from volcanic soil, mixed with lime and interspersed with other materials, often broken tile, according to Glancey. This concrete enabled the Romans to create large domes and huge aqueducts that carried water for miles in the European countryside. Rome had many examples of buildings and statues solely for civic beauty that were durable as well as attractive.

Many examples of architecture on the grand scale were found in the Middle Ages and beyond in the huge cathedrals built in Europe to create emotions of awe and wonder as people contemplated spiritual matters in these beautiful, grand buildings. A fine example is the Cathedral of Notre Dame in Paris, France.

From the beginnings of creating basic shelter, then temples, then architecture for its own sake, come all the building arts. These arts include carpentry, metal working, plastering, brick laying, and many others; not to mention the different methods of beautifying these buildings with mosaics, painting, tile, stained glass, and statuary.

The Power of Pottery

Like construction, pottery is another good example of a hands-on art. The potter manually transforms a mound of clay into an artwork which uses different skills than the visual arts of drawing and painting. It takes feel to center the clay and feel to see if it is symmetrical.

Pottery is another ancient art. Matter of fact, pottery has the same age as civilization. When humans were hunter-gatherers, the container of choice was the woven basket. It was only with the beginning of civilization, agriculture, and a stationary life-style, that pottery became the container of choice to hold grains, seeds, oils, and wine, says Tony Birkes in *The Complete Potter's Guide*. The art of basketry changed to pottery as the need arose.

Sometimes the transition from basketry to pottery was a gradual one. The Indians of the American Southwest first began making baskets that they covered with clay to make them watertight, writes Leroy Appleton in *American Indian Design and Decoration*. There was a gradual transition from baskets, to baskets covered with clay, to eventual pottery. Corn, the main agricultural crop to American Indians, required pottery for storage.

American Indians, like the Greeks, never used the potter's wheel. The process of pottery making varied according to locality, says Appleton. Vessels were sometimes shaped in a mold—usually a basket—or modeled free hand, worked out from a block of clay and beaten into shape with a paddle. Usually, however, the potter used the coil method, where the potter rolls the clay into a long, round rope and then coils it up and smooths the sides together to make a seamless pot. Interestingly enough, Indian women made most of the pottery, says Appleton.

Clay, the material from which pottery is made, is weathered, decomposed granite which is mainly alumina and silica. It has very fine particles which create a very smooth texture. Because of its composition, clay will withstand extreme heat, so it can be heated in a kiln to create a very strong surface. It is very durable after the second firing.

There are two main types of pottery: earthenware and stoneware. These two types vary on the temperature of the second firing when glazing the pot. Earthenware is fired to between 1,800 degrees F to 2,000 degrees F. Most stoneware is fired for the second time between 2,280 degrees F and 2,370 Degrees F. At this temperature the clay itself begins to change and vitrify to make a stronger surface on the piece of pottery.

The potter's primary enjoyment is to be able to take clay, earth from the planet, and simply feel the texture of it. Clay has to be kneaded to make certain that it is homogeneous throughout with no air bubbles. It is an enormously gratifying feeling for the potter to take a lump of earth, change it by way of the potter's wheel or by hand, into something beautiful and useful.

Glazing, the process of putting color onto the clay, requires a good eye and a good imagination. The glazes are not the same colors before and after they are fired. The potter needs to imagine what the glazes will look like before he fires them since he cannot tell the colors that the glazes will ultimately turn. For instance, a color that is somewhat grey may turn out to be a nice green after it is fired. A fired, glazed pot has a nice feel to it. It is pleasant to run the hands over the finished pot just for the pleasure of the shape and the feel of the surface. Pottery has the striking characteristics of being both decorative and useful, economic or extravagant.

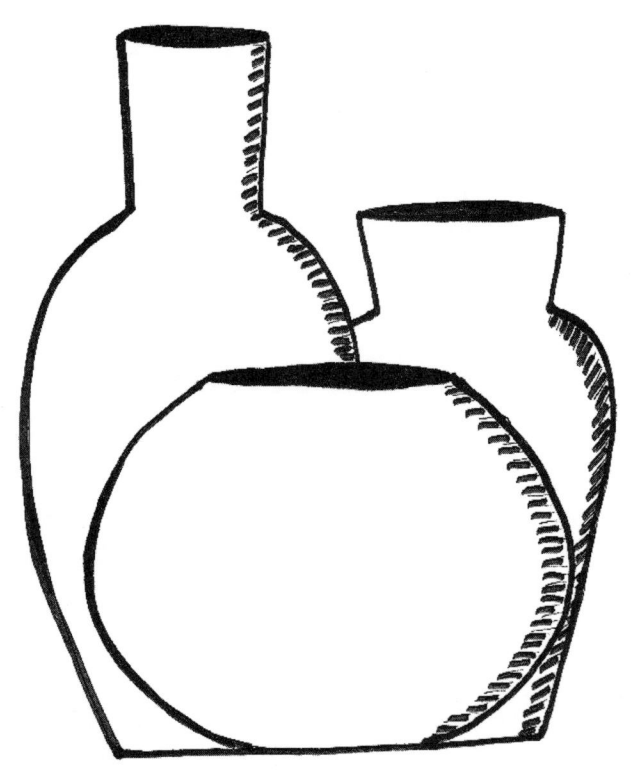

Physical Movement as Art and Mental Stimulation

Physical movement is astonishingly necessary to the workings of the brain. It is probable that the area of the brain for physical movement and the area for emotions evolved concurrently because they are intertwined and adjacent in the brain, says John Ratey, in *A User's Guide to the Brain.* Many emotions are played out as physical movement.

For instance, the heart beats quicker when the person is emotionally aroused. The fight, love, flight or hunger mechanisms are all emotionally charged and ready to produce instant action. Many people attempt to make a distinction between mental and physical stimulation. In reality, there is no difference because whatever the body does is essentially a duality of electrical and chemical processes.

A part of the brain is reserved for eye-hand movements. A person uses this brain center to reach for something, hold, or move an object. This area of the brain is vital for the arts using hand movement; for humans, like other primates, are built to learn from imitation. This brain center acts when the person watches another person performing an activity. The same brain areas are active during observation as during the actual performance of the activity. Thus direct, observational learning happens, says John Allman in *Evolving Brains*.

Dance

Dance, an art form that has developed to combine repetitive, expressive movements with melody and percussion, is one of the oldest arts in the human repetoire. Every tribe and civilization has some musical instrument to create music for dance, from rudimentary instruments such as flute and drum to sophisticated electronic synthesizers. Often dance music is different from other music because it emphasizes rhythm more than melody. In fact, some dance music is just pure rhythm and may be performed solely on drums.

Dance is physical movement ritualized to an art form because the movements are often stylized, symbolic, and can be used to induce emotions and tell stories. Ancient dance was often connected with special events. Hunters danced before the hunt, warriors danced before battle, and the whole tribe danced to please the gods. There were dances to celebrate the harvest, honor a wedding couple, and mourn the dead. Dance connected the tribe with the supernatural as in the Rain Dance that was designed to bring rain.

Even before dance became more highly choreographed, every group of people had rhythmic movements such as swaying, stepping, jumping, stamping, and running that were routinely performed in the community. Each country has dance movements that are highly specialized and characteristic. There are Greek line dances,

Scots highland dancing, and vigorous Russian folk dances. Dancing plays a role in national identity.

Although the beginning of dance was ritualistic and often religious in nature, it quickly was enjoyed for its own sake. There are two main types of dance: the dances that are meant for everyone and may mark some social occasion and those that are meant to be watched by spectators as formal entertainment. In modern society, there is social dancing for everyone, then there is formal, classical ballet where everyone watches and only the ballet company participates. Ballet tells a story whereas social dancing is for group enjoyment.

There are certain skills that are associated with dance. Dance teaches a person to move gracefully, efficiently, and rhythmically. Rhythm is invigorating or relaxing to the human depending on the speed and type of rhythm. The heart, a percussion instrument itself, tries to match the rhythm that it hears.

Dance teaches control of different muscles of the body that are sometimes not routinely used, for dance requires exotic movements that are not in the usual human repetoire. Dance teaches balance. For instance, the ability to turn a pirouette in ballet uses balance and muscles in ways different from normal, everyday activities. Dance requires more intricate balance and timing than walking or running. Stylistic dancing such as ballet is strenuous and requires great flexibility, endurance, strength, timing, coordination, and practice.

Couple dancing enjoys great popularity because it fills a number of different roles for the individual. It also requires special sets of skills. Couple dancing requires the ability to work together and anticipate or direct the moves of a partner. Not only does the person have to know where his own body is in space, time, and sequence, but he also has to anticipate the movement and sequence of his partner. The lead in a couple has to coordinate movements and direct them so that feet do not get tangled, timing does not get off, the sequence is comfortable and doable, and both dancers have a good time. The follower has to remain flexible and anticipate the moves of the lead, and be able to carry out these operations. It requires split-second timing and decision making. The lead gets to plan in advance while the follower has to make split second decisions with no advance notice.

According to research done by Richard Powers, a dancing instructor at Stanford University, the follower gets the most benefit from couple dancing because she makes the most decisions and get the biggest brain workout. Powers quotes a 21-year study of senior citizens by the Albert Einstein College of Medicine in New York City which found that frequent dancing was the activity that gave the most benefit to senior citizens and provided the best defense against Altzheimer's. Ballroom dancing provided a 76% reduction in the onset of Altzheimer's according to this study. Obviously, dancing is a skill that everyone should enjoy into old age.

Dancing is a set of skills that includes many different types of stimuli: There is social contact in couple dancing, physical movement and the enjoyment of music and rhythm. There is the mental challenge of learning new steps where the dancer learns mentally and physically how to maneuver a new sequence. He makes new decisions. Thus, dance provides the participant with mental challenge, an escape from everyday stress, and the opportunity for fitness and relaxation.

Sometime dance is used for specific purposes. For instance, many societies have traditional male dances that are very beautiful, strong, and interesting. In traditional Hungary the soldiers were skilled dancers. When it came time to get recruits for the army, the experienced soldiers would come to town, start some fantastic, enticing dancing and get the young men all stirred up by the excitement of the music, the folk dancing and mellowed with alcohol. The next morning the village youth would find themselves enrolled in the army. Dance is a stirring activity that serves many different purposes for the human in society.

Sports as Art

People transform many common activities into arts. For instance, the common activities of running, walking, and jumping are not art. But, karate, throwing a spear, sword fighting, ice skating, and some other sports are very artistic. Some sports are as artistic as dance.

Sports were originally designed to keep the hunter, soldier in top shape and to keep combat and hunting skills in top form when these skills were not being actively used. This was especially important because humans are extremely vulnerable without some tool or weapon. Sports helped the warriors and hunters to survive.

Sports and dance are similar in that they both concern carefully controlled movement, yet sports are usually for competition and dance is usually for beauty and symbolic content. Dance is performed to music while sports are executed to the roar of thousands of spectators and pumping adrenaline.

An additional benefit from sports is that it often promotes calmness and calm thinking. A repetitive action like swimming or running allows the athlete time to ponder life's problems without anxiety. Sports reduce the stresses in our lives and help iron out the kinks produced by sitting in offices and working on computers or performing other tedious office or factory work.

Physical activity dramatically increases the blood flow to the brain and help the entire body to achieve good overall circulation. Good circulation helps all the organs in the body to function at maximum capacity. Movement, including both dance and sports, has served mankind faithfully in promoting the welfare of the entire mind and body. These are some of the benefits received from sports:

- Sports make a person feel better and become more fit. It adds spring to the step, for moving well is a joy in itself. The sports person feels more relaxed, better able to concentrate, more prone to create. Exercise causes a sense of well-being and energy. Exercise is especially important to those with sedentary lifestyles.

- The knowledge that a person is skilled adds confidence. This confidence influences the attitude of the person in all areas of his life.

- Team and group efforts play a special role in the benefits that can be obtained from sports. Many people believe that they have learned the benefits of working together through sports programs which teach individual and group coordination and cooperation.

- Sports can act as a means to release aggressive, combative, competitive or purely stressful emotions in a controlled atmosphere. This is especially helpful for young men.

Our ability to achieve mental well-being through physical exercise has a long history. John Allman in *Evolving Brains* explains the relationship between serotonin and exercise. The origin of the serotonin system of pleasure centers in the brain is very ancient; it started about 500 million years ago and has been amazingly conserved throughout evolution, says Allman. Serotonin plays an important role in our ability to integrate behavior. Our sense of well-being, the capacity to organize our lives, and the ability to relate to others depends profoundly on the serotonin system. This serotonin system is very small, writes Allman. Only about one millionth of the total population of neurons in the human central nervous system are devoted to this system.

The serotonin system works to keep a delicate balance in nerve activity throughout the central nervous system. This increase in serotonin activity occurs just before physical movement and is apparently driven by the action of the muscles. Physical activity plays a large role in our mental, physical, and chemical balance. Fitness gives energy to our creative spirit.

Spirituality and the Arts

Spirituality is sometimes considered the feeling of being at one with the universe. Sharon Begley in *Newsweek* reports that Dr. James Austin, a neurologist, had discovered that certain parts of the brain must go quiet in order for a human to experience a spiritual moment. The area which checks the world for threats and fear must be damped (amygdala). The area which orients the human in space and marks the distinction between self and the rest of the world must go quiet (frontal and temporal lobe circuits.) Some forms of meditation, prayer, other religious rituals, and the arts do indeed quiet these two branches of the brain. The human then feels afloat in space and at one with the universe.

The arts are often recognized as part of the spiritual process. Almost every religion has stories, music, and visual art. The arts can act much like meditation in that the arts can make the person feel as though he or she is on a different plane of existence and in the mood to contemplate those concepts that are larger than life: the profound.

Much of art is specifically designed to stimulate this feeling of larger-than-life. For instance, the large cathedrals in Europe were designed with the specific intent of providing awe to those who entered these magnificent buildings and encourage them to contemplate spiritual matters.

The contemplation of beauty also sends the human to a different plane of existence. For example, the temples of Greece or the statues of Rodin encourage us to view life in a grand manner and rise above our common, everyday interpretations of life.

The arts connect us spiritually to those who went before us. Contemplating the arts of the great artists and creators of the past lets us realize that we still understand what they were trying to say even though eons have passed. We can observe the spirit of those who have lived before us still and see that they still exist by means of their art works. The Great Pyramind and the Sphinx in Egypt continue to fill us all with wonder at the accomplishments of these people long past. These works of art connect us. We can see that what we and our civilizations do can have an impact on those that follow. We can leave our footprints on the sands of time.

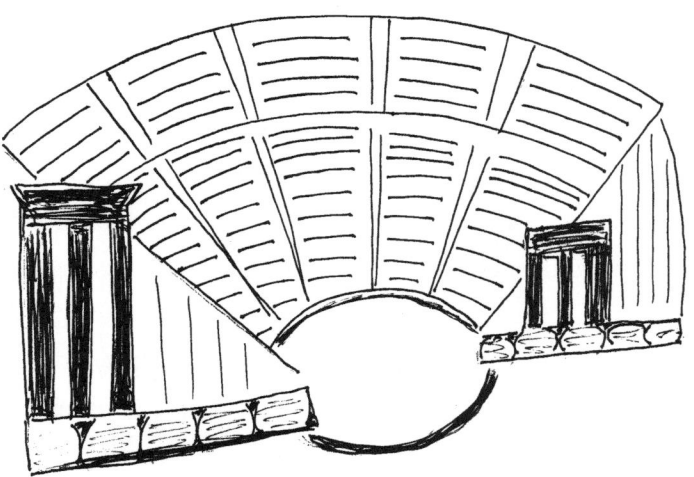

QUESTIONS TO CONSIDER

1. WHAT SORT OF MUSIC MOVES YOU?

2. DO YOU ENJOY DANCING TO MUSIC? WHAT KIND?

3. DO YOU EXERCISE, DO SPORTS TO RELIEVE STRESS AND IMPROVE YOUR MENTAL OUTLOOK? HOW?

4. DO YOU SURROUND YOURSELF WITH BEAUTY? WHAT KIND?

5. HAVE YOU TRIED TO LEARN AN ART FORM FROM IMITATION? WAS IT SUCCESSFUL?

6. HOW OFTEN DO YOU GO TO THE ART GALLERY?

7. DO YOU PLAY A MUSICAL INSTRUMENT? WHICH ONE?

Chapter IX

MENTAL STIMULATION, QUALITY AND LENGTH OF LIFE

A person cannot be happy and well adjusted without a steady stream of mental stimulation. Some people are content to express themselves in calm pursuits like the arts and sports, while others need to jump long distances on motorcycles like Evil Knieval, ride the race cars at a professional racetrack, or even turn to drugs and alcohol for their stimulation. A human will seek stimulation in one way or another, preferably in positive ways that are not unnecessarily harmful to the individual or others. The arts provide benign mental stimulation.

Some of the problems that people face in modern society are the need to start over, deal with crises, and cope with continual everyday stress. Whether it be changes in family, sickness, birth, death, divorce, or natural calamity, job strife, being fired, finding a new job, moving to a new home; people start over several times during their lives. A brain that has been mentally stimulated and educated has a greater variety of choices to choose from when confronted with the array of challenging problems.

The stimulated brain is the flexible brain. Flexibility is the key to survival. Matter of fact, the large brain was developed precisely to deal with fluctuations in the environment. Our environment still fluctuates.

The stimulated, educated, creative brain does not have to be trained at the university. A person can keep learning and keep her mind active through other methods such as the getting information from the internet, reading, talking with others, learning from others, going to public lectures and workshops, and creating.

The stimulated, active brain has more flexible mechanisms to repair memory. Stimulation aids in brain repair, says Ronald Kotulak in *Inside the Brain*. Those who have used their brains their whole lives will enjoy the benefits of mental adaptability when times get tough. The stimulated brain has more neurons and more chance of rebuilding in case of injury or old age. A well-used brain comes with many advantages.

Mental stimulation enhances the flow of blood to the brain causing the brain to stay in better physical condition. Education, i.e. mental stimulation, has been seen as a way to prevent Alzheimer's disease.

The high tech world is changing so quickly that humans must adapt to a new world every time a new technology is developed. Life has become fast paced and mentally complex. Mental stimulation sometimes seems so pervasive in our fast-paced world that it becomes a stressor. Mental flexibility and agility to face continual changes during the human lifetime, the lengthened human life span, continue to be criteria for survival. The stimulated, flexible brain is vital; by means of mental stimulation, the wise person devises criteria for dealing with crises and continual stressors in his life. Modern life changes more quickly than ever before.

UCLA performed autopsies on university graduates who had remained mentally active throughout their lives, and they had 40 percent more brain connections than high school dropouts, says Kotulak in *Inside the Brain*. That by itself should be one stimulus to go to the university, simply to feed the brain. A lack of education in life limits the possibilities of the individual. Seventy five percent of all imprisoned males in America have poor school records and low IQ's and did not grow up with both parents, says Kotulak. The level of education, i.e. mental stimulation, is one of the best indicators of long life in the United States. Educated people (or anyone who keeps learning), says Kotulak, age better because they have several advantages:

- A higher standard of living. They live in better areas with less crime, less pollution, and generally better conditions for life.

- Lack of many chronic diseases because of better diet. Those with education will read the literature and try to prevent heart disease and other ailments caused by diet. They might also head for the organic section at the grocery store instead of the Twinkies. "The rapid rise in the educational level of Americans was reflected in the ability of many people to inform themselves to a far greater extent than ever before about health matters, says Cousins.

- Activity in reading, travel, culture, education, clubs and professional associations. Those people who keep more active in all areas have a better chance of receiving continual and better quality mental stimulation. This variety of activities acts as a buffer against the array of stressors in the society, provides social contact, and gives the person a break from stress.

- Willingness and ability to change. Educated people have already spent years changing their ideas as they gain more information into how they might want to live their lives. As a result, they see more alternatives in any one crisis. Education shows more possibilities and gives the person more choices when it comes time to make a decision.

- Probable marriage to a smart spouse. It is good to surround oneself with positive, intelligent, productive people. Negative, rigid people should be avoided at all costs.

- The ability to grasp new ideas. The educated person has had more practice grasping new ideas though educational experience. As society requires these people to learn yet another skill, it is a manageable task.

- More strenuous activity, exercise, which improves blood flow and oxygen flow to the brain. As the motor and mental systems are so closely connected, within a normal range, what is good for one is good for the other. An educated person has received more mental stimulation by way of more physical stimulation during his or her life.

- The belief that what the individual does makes a difference in his life: personal satisfaction. The value of believing that what the individual does is vital to emotional and mental well-being. As social animals, people are content when they feel that they are doing good for the community, humanity, or the world as a whole.

As to the future of the human brain, it remains to be seen what will happen. Surprisingly, the human brain is shrinking. The domesticated dog has a brain that is about three quarters the size of the wolf of equivalent body size and weight. The fact that the dog is domesticated has caused his brain to shrink because he is no longer a predator but a couch potato who receives supper out of a can. Along those same lines, the human brain has lost size in the last 35,000 years, writes John Allman in *Evolving Brains*. Through our invention of agriculture, cities, and domesticated plants and animals for our food supply, we have domesticated ourselves and must pay the price.

The brain is far more changeable and delicately balanced than was ever suspected. It was found that flight attendants who worked for long periods of time on airplanes and went across several time zones were noticing mental changes. The data reveal that jet lag without sufficient recovery time between trips affects the brain's structure and function, writes a journalist for The Washington Post. There are many delicate nuances of brain function that are still not known or understood.

In the future, humanity will adapt to the artificial world we have created where our flexible minds will be stretched to the limit. A survival advantage in the past may become detrimental in contemporary life. For example, sedentary life-styles and a following reduction in the activation of the serotonin system may be responsible for increased levels of psychological problems in modern society, writes Allman. Dealing with our past adaptations and wondering how we will evolve in the future is a continuous process. The brain needs constant learning, care, tending, and creative expression. Taking care of the human brain by way of mental stimulation, especially in the arts, is a life-long project. Use it or lose it; but use it wisely.

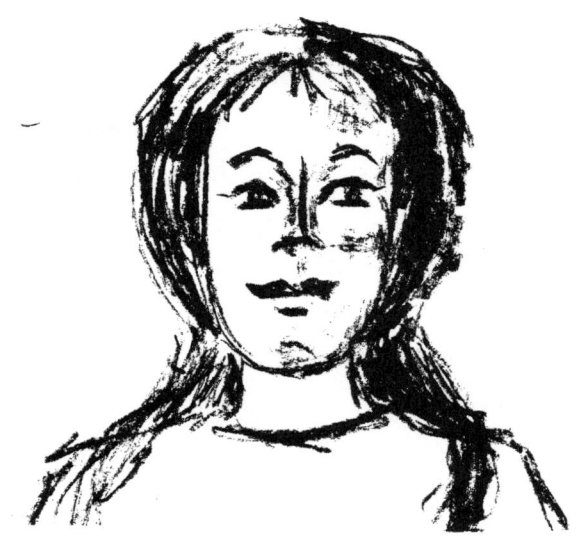

QUESTIONS TO CONSIDER

1. DO YOU BELIEVE THAT YOU GET ENOUGH STIMULATION AND LEARNING TO KEEP YOUR BRAIN ALIVE?

2. AS A LIFE-LONG PROJECT, HOW CAN YOU MAXIMIZE YOUR LEARNING AND MENTAL STIMULATION?

3. WHAT NEW ACTIVITIES AND CHALLENGES WAIT IN YOUR FUTURE?

4. HOW CAN YOU BALANCE YOUR NEED FOR STIMULATION WITH THE NEED TO EARN A LIVING?

5. DO YOU SET AN EXAMPLE FOR OTHERS? HOW?

6. CAN YOU SHARE YOUR ARTISTIC EXPRESSION WITH OTHER PEOPLE? IF SO, HOW?

7. HAS THIS BOOK BEEN HELPFUL TO YOUR THINKING ABOUT THE HEALTH OF THE HUMAN BRAIN AS IT RELATES TO THE ARTS? (See address in the front pages of the book to send reply.)

Epilogue

Working to Keep an Active, Balanced Brain

Simple Everyday Activities for the Brain

Richard Restak in *Mozart's Brain and the Fighter Pilot,* lists many common, everyday activities that are good for the upkeep of the brain, and which do not require a lot of equipment or preplanning. These can be done by everyone. His list is broken down into three categories:

• *Passive Activities* which include social clubs, church get togethers, talking on the phone, or visiting someone in person, and listening to music. Except for music, these are social activities which promote brain health.

• *Intellectual Activities* which include reading, doing puzzles, playing music, doing crafts and artwork, writing, playing games, sewing and needlework, and even buying groceries without using a list. Playing demanding games like chess and bridge are beneficial to the individual. Not only are these games mentally demanding but they also provide social contact at the same time. The brain requires work and stimulation.

- *Physical Activities* include sports, working out in the gym, bicycling, gardening, skating, swimming, and walking. Apparently, a special emphasis can be placed on ballroom dancing which provides lifelong benefits.

Relaxing activities that still require the person to make decisions and stay alert are beneficial, even such simple activities as driving in the country on a Sunday afternoon. It is especially stimulating to drive to a new area, which requires that the driver notice new signs, new turns, read the map, find a new place for lunch, and discover the different possibilities in new towns or places that the driver has never been. Any common activity that requires brain work is great.

Hiking, skiing, camping, canoeing and all the other activities that allow the person to be out of doors, into natural scenic areas, and doing activity that is physically demanding is therapeutic. The brain that was adapted for the African savannah enjoys a break from city life once in a while. Being out in the natural world is good for the eyes, because the eyes get tired of focusing up close for computer work and other work that we do for a living. The opportunity to gaze into the distance, see the valleys, and see the sunset are a nice vacation for the eyes. The quietness of the wood, with just the birds singing in the brush, is a nice break from the sirens, traffic, helicopters, rock music, loud movies and other auditory stress that we experience in our everyday lives in the city.

As previously stated, art projects or any other projects or areas of personal or professional interest keep the mind actively occupied. Creative work strengthens the brain. Many people have jobs that let them make decisions, create, work with others, solve problems, mediate between worker disputes, advise, critique, create a good product, work with the public, or provide customer service. These skills keep the brain active as long as the work does not become so long or so intense that it becomes a stressor rather than a pleasant stimulus. Useful work is important to our lives.

The Role of Positive Thinking

Restak further emphasizes that the brain is an accumulation of the thoughts that the individual thinks. Thinking makes the brain. Like the athlete who visualizes the perfect jump before winning the Gold Medal at the Olympics, so each person must visualize what he or she wants to happen. If the individual dwells on anxiety, depression, or negative thoughts, these will become the individual's reality. Consequently, positive thinking plays a big role in keeping the brain fit and smoothly functioning.

Diet and Mind Enhancing drugs

Diet itself plays a central role in the successful operation of the brain and its creativity. There are the usual dietary guidelines of not overeating, not eating too much fat or salt. However, the brain does need some of these items. It is recommended to watch blood pressure and cholesterol levels in order to hinder the incidence of stroke. Basically, the diet that is good for the heart is also good for the brain. That diet is one full of a great variety of fruits and vegetables to get all the different nutrients and a diet that is lower on meat products. Yet, protein is also important. The question of carbohydrates such, as bread and pasta, is currently up for debate. Some say that we need carbohydratess for fuel for exercise, while others say that carbohydrates are not that necessary.

People will augment their mental capacities with mind enhancing drugs. The term "smart drugs" came into existence in 1991 with the publication of *Smart Drugs and Nutrients*, says Ward Dean, author of *Smart Drugs*. A smart drug is any drug or nutrient which enhances some aspect of mental performance. Smart drugs can be anything from vitamins to gingko biloba. The American public, interested in brain enhancement and retention, is now using more nutritional supplements than ever before. Americans spend $3.3 billion on vitamins and nutrients every year, says Dean, and that figure is growing. Taking some kind of supplements is now mainstream healthcare.

We are at a similar place with smart drugs as we were 10 years ago with vitamins. We're a few years away from them becoming part of our consensus reality, says Dean. A common example of a smart drug is the caffeine in coffee. With the aging of the baby boomers, those born soon after World War II, a lot of thought is being spent on the subject of prolonging good health and deferring the problems of aging. The baby boomers don't want to get old. The younger generation doesn't want them to age either, because they don't want to pay for their care. The baby boomers are emphasizing preventative health, of which smart drugs is one of the components. However, smart drugs can enhance the performance of the younger person as well as raise the quality of life for the elderly.

Catering to the baby boomers is big business. According to the *Economist*, "the American Pharmaceutical industry is developing more than 140 types of smart pills in its laboratories, making them the tenth-largest class of drugs being researched." says Dean. Since the baby boomers are such a large group, their health and aging is a national concern.

Joseph Coates in his article "Brain Technology on Way" in *Research Management Today* speaks about new drugs for brain management. For example, he claims Prozac is "the closest thing to a make you feel good, make you perform better pill. Prozac is just the opening wedge on families of new drugs. . ." The future for new brain enhancers is on the way.

The use of smart drugs is very individual. This means that enough is enough, too little won't do anything, and too much will have the opposite effect from what the person is expecting, says Dean. Only the individual with the help of a physician can determine what is the right dose of smart drugs and nutrients. It depends on the size of the person, weight, metabolism, age and other variables. It takes a certain amount of trial and error to find the exact amount that works.

In 1988, a California research team headed by Dr. Stephen Schoenthaler and the English research team of Benton and Roberts both found that giving school children simple vitamin supplements produced a nonverbal IQ increase of an average of six points, says Dean.

Not all the students showed an increase in IQ; however, one third of them had a ten-point jump which suggests that about 30 percent of the children suffer from a vitamin deficiency in their diet. An earlier study by Sandstead (1986) and Cherkin (1987) found that mental dysfunction is one of the first effects of nutritional deficiency and dietary problems. Even small lacks of vital elements can cause pronounced effects.

Lack of the correct nutrients can be especially vital for the person in a weaker position, namely the young and the elderly. It is easy to see the correlation between mental disfunction and certain vitamins and minerals. Here is a brief list of some nutrients and what possible effects may be caused by their lack.

Vitamin	Effect
B1, Thiamine	Beri beri, Psychosis
B2, Riboflavin	Cognitive impairment, memory deficit
B3, Niacin	Pellaga, dementia, rage
B5, Pantothenic acid	Myelin degeneration
B6, Pyridoxine	Convulsions, peripheral neuropathy
B12, Cobalamin	Dementia, peripheral neuropathy, sub-acute combined system degeneration, cognitive impairment, memory deficit, depression, parethesia, ataxia, mood disturbances, delusions, paranoia
Folate, folic acid	irritability, depression, paranoia, cognitive impairment, memory

	deficit, forgetfulness, EEG abnormalities, dementia, epilepsy, schizophrenia
Vitamin C, ascorbate	cognitive impairment, memory deficit
Vitamin E, tocopherol	Peripheral axonopathy, spinocereballar degeneration

Almost any vitamin and nutrient deficiency can cause cognitive impairment, says Dean. These deficiencies are most common in the elderly. The deficiencies of Vitamin B12, folic acid, and vitamin B6 are responsible for much of the mental impairment observed in elderly individuals. It can easily be corrected through nutritional supplements. Deficiencies in hydrochloric acid, (HCL), the acid that breaks down foods in the stomach for digestion can diminish the ability of the body to absorb vitamins. Thirty percent of the elderly, 65 and over, have a serious problem with digestion. Many of the vitamins cannot be restored to the normal level with the RDA (recommended daily amount) of the vitamin. Correcting an existing deficiency was not taken into account when the RDA amounts were determined, says Dean.

On the other hand, people who take certain supplements may find that they are adversely affected. The overdose of some vitamin or mineral may cause heart palpitations, allergies, or other unpleasant side effects. The individual should proceed cautiously when adding any supplements to the diet.

Diet, especially for some people, can be crucial in preventing depression. Some people who have a strong reaction to sugar can become depressed after they ingest sugar and the brief burst of pleasure and energy wears off. The depression can make them crave another boost of energy, so the person runs out to get another candy bar. This can be a huge problem for people who are overweight. It is an addiction. Robert Thayer, in *The Origin of Everyday Moods,* mentions a study that proved that "diets from which sugar has been eliminated lead to decreases in depression."

Dean says that the effects of vitamins and minerals, much like other drugs, operate on the inverse bell curve also, with each individual having to find his own correct dosage. The FDA has traditionally claimed that amino acids, herbs, and high potency vitamins are toxic, says Dean. These items are toxic only if taken in an amount that is not correct for the individual. If the individual determines the correct dosage of a vitamin or mineral, his personal nutrition and brain function may be enhanced as he receives extra nutrients that he individually needs in greater or lessor amounts than others. Those who do not eat right or cannot absorb nutrients run the risk of losing brain function unnecessarily.

Dealing With Sensory Deprivation

In times of sensory deprivation, such as divorce, death of a loved one, depression, boring jobs, or aging; the individual must make an effort to seek out mental stimulation, social contact, and the means to process any current problems.

Linda Richman in *I'd Rather Laugh* solved her feelings of grief at the death of her son by staging what she calls a "pity party." Because the brain begins to put into the background any stimulus that it continually receives in large amounts, the pity party is designed to inundate the brain with pity. Richman listened to sad music, watched sad movies, just generally wallowed in sadness for two days. Then the third day, it is back to the normal business of living. She allowed herself to feel pain but only for a controlled, finite period.

Richman further suggests that people pay attention to their flags, the signals that tell them when they are in distress. They may be headaches, depression, sickness, exhaustion, anxiety attacks, recurrent colds, allergies, or any other sign that the person needs to be especially careful with feelings and deal with them. To ignore these signs is a serious mistake. People must deal with these problems and help themselves reach a state of equilibrium when something has put them out of balance. When something is wrong, they must act to fix it before the problem becomes too big to handle.

Some of the lifelong consequences of grieving include periodic bouts of recurring emotions brought up by an event that triggers strong memories of the deceased. A certain place, piece of music, or holiday will suddenly remind one of the person who is gone. As a result, the person is never completely free of remembering the grief he experienced. Time must pass to lessen the wounds of the mourner. However, death is not the only situation to cause grief.

Most people finds themselves more spiritual after the death of a loved one which manifests itself in different ways. Some start to feel greater emotion in the presence of beauty from art or music, for instance. Some people become more religious while others will find themselves more interested in nature and taking a walk in the woods. Many start to ponder the great questions of the universe, while others show the desire to help people like themselves in the grieving condition. Death deeply affects our spiritual side and makes us think in a whole new way.

Psychologists worry about someone who says he has no reactions to a death, is carrying on as if nothing happened, or is being strong and will not let himself grieve. Avoidance of the process is not beneficial because grief must be dealt with, if not now, then later, but it will happen. A person has to mourn. It may be through the arts, through helping others, through solitude, through prayer, that the grieving person finally works through the pain.

Sometimes life's events take a toll on us mentally. A writer who was taking a class in writing experienced writers block upon the deaths of both her parents. She went into shock and found that her creativity went dormant during her extreme emotional crisis. The condition was not permanent. Fortunately, creativity came back when the trauma and the loss began to subside about three to four years later.

Art excels at providing manageable short-term goals for the griever. It provides something positive to do during mourning, even if creativity is down. Many arts require extreme concentration which prevent the mind from thinking on negative thoughts. Making an attempt at anything creative starts the mind thinking in a more positive direction.

Another negative circumstance is depression. One antidote to mild depression caused by a temporary situation is to make decisions in order to feel in control of life. Helplessness, hoplessness, and lack of direction are just some of the traps that the mildly depressed can fall into. Just making a decision, any decision, is a critical first step to recovery.

Since humans are, to a certain extent, in control of their reality, they can make conscious decisions not to wander down the road to depression. The optimist who thinks positively is less likely to become depressed than the pessimist who concentrates on the negative. However, this does not mean that the person should not feel negative emotions and accept them for what they are, just part of life.

The single most important factor that appears to protect people from negative moods is education (i.e. mental stimulation), says behavioral scientist Bruce S. Jonas of the National Center for Health Sciences, as quoted by Kotulak in *Inside the Brain*. The person with education sees many different options and choices of action for any situation and is more likely to seek stimulation.

Often a brain that is sinking into depression is suffering from a lack of stimulation. If the brain is not busy, it starts to get out of balance. Anything that puts the brain to work in a positive direction is beneficial. A content brain is not bored or unused.

In the attempt to find stimulation, the individual must beware of what kind of stimulation he finds. When the individual is feeling down, negative aspects of daily life should be avoided, such as the evening news. As newspaper people say: If it bleeds, it leads. The media is looking for shocking events to attract attention not to be cheerful. The news on TV or the newspaper can help to keep a person in a negative, fearful, anxious frame of mind and dampen attempts to feel positive and work for a brighter future. On the other hand, it is good for the individual to have an idea of what is happening in the world. Being totally unaware is not good. There is a fine balance people walk to maintain mental equilibrium.

Another antidote for depression is to keep busy. The person who is not employed and has nothing to do should make up something. There is always a new adventure waiting. The arts and exercise work wonders.

Thayer reports the outcome of a Gallup poll in 1986. When asked what people did to relieve depression, (a) 77 percent reported spending more time alone with a hobby, TV, reading or listening to music, (b) 68 percent said seeking out friends to talk with, (c) 66 percent said seeking out family members to talk with, and (d) 64 percent said raising or lowering the amount that they ate to alleviate depression.

The depressed person or the mourner has to come to grips with the situation and decide what he wants to do. He can either live in hopelessness, fear, and anxiety or get out there and seize the day. The choice is up to the individual.

No matter what direction the depressed person heads, it is a difficult problem to handle. For those who are lightly depressed by life's events, self help may be enough to break it. For those who are deeply and clinically depressed by chemical imbalances; doctors, psychotherapy and medications may be a necessity.

The Need for Social Contact

A main ingredient in our lives and our survival is the desire for human social contact. The early humans adapted to life in small communal groups of about twenty-five people. These groups hunted and raised children together. They stayed together for protection, learned together, and defended themselves as a group. Different people in the group took on different jobs, thus allowing for role and job diversity. The whole basis of human existence is built upon the cooperation of the group not just lone humans living independently. People work together to succeed as a species.

Humans evolved as part of a large extended family which modern society has changed. With humans being so mobile and with jobs changing so quickly, people are always on the move. Modern life in the United States is too isolating to be beneficial to the species. The present mode of living is against history, against human nature, and causes stresses which take an enormous toll on the productivity of the society.

Employees now work on machines and computers which cause further isolation. They communicate with each other through computers in the high tech age. Humans are isolated and alienated from their group, from each other. They miss the sense of belonging and working together for a common goal that was prevalent in life in smaller groups.

To add to this isolation are many single-parent families with children or single people living by themselves. Divorce deprives the parents and children of an extended family and the sense of continuity, belonging, or security that existed in previous generations.

People must have social contact, without which brain cells start to die. People in isolation have three times more chance of dying of heart disease. One study found that group psychotherapy before surgery doubled the post-surgical life-span of women with breast cancer, says Thomas Lewis in *A General Theory of Love*.

Human contact is necessary for the elderly and those in hospitals. Often they are ignored by family and medical staff, both of whom are too busy to give them much time. Norman Cousins, in *Anatomy of an Illness*, writes that hospital patients fear the "utter void created by the longing—ineradicable, unremitting, pervasive—for warmth of human contact. A warm smile and an outstretched hand were valued even above the offering of modern science, but the latter were far more accessible than the former." When the person needs personal contact the most is when he or she will least receive it. Formerly this contact was provided by the extended family.

The uniquely human feature that differentiates us from other primates is our ability to participate in a large variety of different social networks, each with its own rights and obligations, says Allman. Because we participate in such a variety of groups: work groups, economic groups, social groups, exercise groups, it is impossible to state a size of the human social group in modern society.

Matter of fact, our need for social contact has even extended across species. For instance, the domestication of the dog occurred approximately 135,000 years ago, says Allman. This partnership of dog and human has been present in almost all societies on earth. This union has added enormous survival advantage to humans because the dog acted as protector and was better able to run down food and all the dog required was a little TLC and a share of the bounty from the hunt. This union between human and pet has proved so beneficial that currently, in most assisted living centers for the elderly, it is acceptable for the senior citizen to retain a beloved pet.

Pets emphasize the difficulty of humans bonding. There are a lot of dangerous humans in any given society, and some people find it easier to bond with a different species, a pet, than to bond with a fellow human. Matter of fact, we use pets to protect us from each other. Humans ultimately fair best who join meaningful social networks to constantly interact with others.

Laughter as Social Contact

It is important to enjoy ourselves and our lives. One way to accomplish this goal is by promoting laughter. Laughter is a very positive influence in our lives. We all know the wonderful effect of a good laugh; it can turn our day from dreary to bright in a few golden moments. Everyone is attracted to the person who has a good sense of humor. Lucky are we who have the good fortune to live with someone who possesses a great sense of humor and has the charisma to use it privately at home in the family setting as well as in more public occasions where it will receive more payback.

The power of laughter is strong medicine. Norman Cousins, in *Anatomy of Illness*, describes how he decided to take his serious illness, a problem with the connective tissues in his body, into his own hands. He asked the questions: "If negative emotions produce negative chemical changes in the body, wouldn't positive emotions produce positive chemical changes? Is it possible that love, hope, faith, laughter, confidence, and the will to live have therapeutic value?" He left the depressing hospital environment and checked into a hotel; he told his family to find jokes and funny videos for him, then he proceeded to fill himself with humor and huge amounts of Vitamin C. By taking his health into his own hands and deciding for himself what would be most beneficial, he became his own best medicine.

Cousins discovered that "Ten minutes of genuine belly laughter had an anesthetic effect and would give me at least two hours of pain-free sleep." By his use of positive stimuli and a positive environment, Cousins overcame his serious illness.

Robert Provine in his book, *Laughter*, studies the biological, evolutionary, and social aspects of laughter. "Biologically speaking, laughter is a basic element of human nature. Birds tweet and humans laugh. Laughter can be regarded as 'human song,' " concludes Provine.

Laughter is an instinctive behavior programmed by our genes. It is a universal human phenomenon, although not all societies agree on what is funny. In spite of laughter being universal and genetic, each person has an individual laugh and an individual sense of humor.

The human need for laughter is no joke, Provine claims. It serves a dual purpose in human social settings, both promoting the bonding of the group as well as humiliating and ostracizing outsiders. Sometimes, laughter is coupled with teasing. Teasing, like laughter, can be enjoyable or used to control people, bring them discomfort, and make them look weak in the face of the attacker.

A good leader uses laughter to relax and unite a group. Terry Kimchuk, speech writer to the Doles, said that Bob Dole often used humor to make the senate work. When Dole stepped into the room with representatives from opposing political parties, and he cracked a few jokes so the group could relax and tackle the work they had come together to accomplish. Kimchuk further mentions that, politically speaking, the most successful presidents are the ones that were outgoing, charismatic, and had an active sense of humor like Lincoln, Kennedy, and Roosevelt.

Every human responds to laughter. Of course, not all societies view laughter in the same manner. Nothing is more difficult than trying to tell a joke in a foreign language, because the speaker quickly discovers that ideas that are funny in one culture are not funny in another.

Laughter is contagious everywhere. When one human sees another laughing, the second begins to laugh along with the first. This raises the intriguing possibility that humans have an auditory laugh-detector, a neural circuit in our brain that responds exclusively to laughter, Provine states. If there were no laugh detector, then how would humans pick up on others laughing? Why do humans collectively laugh? Maybe it is for the comfort of social bonding that takes place and for the health benefits that affect the group as a whole and make the society a better, calmer place. It serves as a way to relieve the stresses that the structure of the group provides.

Each society has certain rules of laughter. For example, it is considered socially unacceptable to laugh at funerals in the United States. However, since laughter is not always under control a socially unapproved episode may occur at times of deep stress; it is possible for an unfortunate mourner to break out in laughter for sheer release. In which case, the mourner ostracizes himself.

Laughter has unique characteristics: for instance, "speakers laugh more than their audiences, women laugh at men more than men laugh at women, and laughter has more to do with relationships than jokes," says Provine. People in more dominant social positions are more likely to deliver humor while those in more dependent roles are more likely to laugh. No one dares to keep a straight face when the boss tells a joke. Laughter helps to establish the social hierarchy.

"Women seek men who make them laugh and men are anxious to comply with this request," states Provine. In testing the health of a relationship, it is the laughter of the women that is important. "Guys can laugh or not, but it's best that their woman is getting her yucks in."

The process of laughter is shared with our nearest relatives the monkeys. Provine says that chimpanzees and apes do not share the same laughter as humans because of breath control. The ape, because it runs on four feet, has to have its lungs full of air to act as a cushion every time all four feet hit the ground. Therefore the ape has to exhale and inhale with every burst of laughter whereas the human can take a huge breath because of upright posture and can laugh for an extended period of time. We potentially owe our ability to have a good laugh to the fact that we stand upright and do not run on all fours.

Laughter fulfills part of the essential human need for mental stimulation by way of social contact. People who laugh together come away rejuvenated and in good spirits.

Practicing Language Skills

Acute language skills are essential to keeping our brains stimulated and our lives running smoothly. When language skills get rusty, people don't fare well at first meeting. It affects people's ability to be social with others. Good language skills promote good communication;

good communication is successful social contact. Successful social contact equals a happy person with a content brain.

Speaking and Storytelling

One way to practice language skills is by creating a story, either written or oral. One of the characteristics that make storytelling of special interest to humans is that it is often symbolic and the human language system thrives on symbolism. Storytelling works best when filled with interesting dialogue, full of description of the characters and the setting, and full of unexpected surprises. In addition, the audience likes to draw their own conclusions not be given the explanation or moral of the story.

Most people fear speaking in public. The way to conquer the fear of public speaking is to deal with the brain on its own terms. The brain has an anxiety attack at public speaking for the first time because it is a novel situation and the brain picks up on the novelty and becomes agitated. The heart speeds up, the mouth becomes dry, the speaker breaks out in a sweat, butterflies form in the stomach, and the speaker stutters nervously.

Since the brain ignores events that become habitual, the first order of business is to make public speaking habitual. The potential speaker should take advantage of every opportunity to do public speaking, from doing presentations at the office to telling the kids stories at bedtime. As soon as the situation is no longer novel, when the speaker rises to speak, the brain will go, "ho, hum, not public speaking again," and remain relaxed. However, a little bit of nervousness makes a better presentation, because a boring speaker is an overly complacent speaker.

The speaker who takes the attitude that he has a message of importance to deliver and wants to share this message with the audience for their benefit will have less stage fright and a more relaxed presentation than the speaker who is trying to be a star. The speaker should be the vehicle for the message or idea not an end in himself.

One means to learn public speaking in a nurturing environment is to join Toastmasters International, a non-profit, public speaking organization. Groups like Toastmasters become progressively more necessary in an age where people are becoming more and more dependent on computers for their communication rather than talking face to face with real humans. Toastmasters gives people the ability to speak directly to each other. There are many different skills to be learned in the field of public speaking:

The speaker gains confidence as he learns that he can speak in front of an audience, or one on one, with poise, dignity and continue to think at the same time. A poor speaker panics to the point that his brain goes into automatic and he loses control over whatever he is saying. The seasoned speaker controls nervousness in order to function normally in front of a group.

Impromptu speaking, speaking without preparation, allows the potential speaker to learn to handle herself with more calmness and poise when called upon to make surprise presentations or answer unexpected questions. A person was coming out of the libary one day, and on the steps was a reporter for the evening news. The reporter asked her a controversial question and she had to make a spontaneous attempt to sound dignified in front of the whole TV audience of her city without previous notice or planning. A little practice in public speaking and the ability to field unexpected questions is a useful skill.

The mental stimulation received from speaking includes the ability to hold the attention of the audience and be able to communicate something during the time the speaker holds audience attention. Speaking and actually connecting with a group is a very powerful experience. The speaker can feel when he connects because the group usually becomes very silent and intense with concentration and anticipation.

Things to do in Drama and Acting

There are many opportunities to join small drama groups and attend their performances. Classes and performances in drama are found at the local community colleges and universities.There is Shakespearean Theater and professional theater with many different types of drama for people to watch and absorb. Books of plays sit on the shelves at the local library which a person can read. A family can even get together and read plays for enjoyment. The action can be videotaped by a friend. There are programs on public TV or radio where a person can get involved with live productions on the media. The world is full of possibilities.

Reading and Writing

In the computer age, average citizens are more likely to record and publish or desk-top publish themselves. Writers can now post works on the internet for others to read without even actually being published in book form. The ability to record our thoughts has added greatly to our ability to learn and has enhanced our ability to remember. We can use our books to give us the details that we don't want to take the time to memorize. The written word, either written by ourselves or read from the writing of others, stimulates the imagination and the brain. Writing remains a useful and necessary skill.

A good idea for writing practice is to keep a diary where the writer records thoughts and works through the problems of the day. Many times, just the act of writing down a problem enables the writer to see the problem with more clarity and reach a conclusion that would have evaded the writer had he not had the courage to write.

Coping Skills

We learn to endure crises with finesse. How to survive when the calamities hit, the sensory deprivations occur, we become older, or we become isolated for one reason or another is the challenge. These are the author's suggestions on mental survival:

Be calm. *Stress is just not worth it.* Stress prevents us from accomplishing our goals. The less we let the little things upset us, the more energy we have to tackle the serious problems in a positive, constructive manner.

Be a lifelong student; *learning keeps us mentally young.* The longer we can keep the mind learning and flexible, the more chance we have to deal with our challenges when they arise. An inflexible, unlearned mind has lost the ability to cope and adapt.

Enjoy your kids and let them go. There is nothing we can do about their leaving anyway. Kids seems to enjoy their parents far more after they have children themselves and look forward to seeing us as grandparents.

Keep a social circle of friends. We age the best when we are socially a part of a group. We cannot expect family to fill in all the gaps in our lives; we need outside friends to talk to, to interact with, and to stimulate us.

Accept infirmities when they arrive; *they cannot be avoided.* We all have to die of some cause. We know from looking at our family tree what to expect. We need to meet those catastrophes with as much grace as possible.

Keep active and eat well. *Keep the blood flow and nutrients supplied to the brain.* Activity and diet goes a long way towards keeping us fit, mentally and physically.

Be eternally willing to start over. Life throws many curves, and every time we have to get up and begin again. If we get an illness, if a loved one leaves or dies, we start over to adapt to that problem. It we move to a new city, we start over to make new friends. We are always adapting to new conditions in one way or another.

Have a sense of self. Our sense of self is probably the one constant throughout our lives. We need to know who we are, what we want, what we will or will not do, what we need, and what we have to offer our friends and community.

Keep a sense of humor. In the end, that is all that we have. Those of us who have a good sense of humor go through life better, have fewer problems both healthwise and psychologically, are much more pleasant to be around when we age, and fare better socially. Humor is a great talent to appreciate in ourselves and others.

Be spiritual. Believing in a greater purpose than oneself is beneficial. A larger view of the universe makes life more inspiring and prevents shortsightedness.

Art and Interests. Any person should always have an art project and some field of particular interest, for fun, for stimulation, and for the joy of creating, learning, and sharing with others.

Appendix I

FUTURE DEVELOPMENTS

Genetically Altered Humans

With the processes now available to genetically alter plants, the technology is quickly coming where humans can be genetically altered, too. Some say that this is the only way to go because evolution is such a slow process that humans will never evolve fast enough to function in our fast, high-tech, modern world. Others say that fiddling with Nature is a dangerous occupation because we do not know the consequences of what we do. For instance, if we start doing our own genetic manipulation, we could ruin the survival qualities of the genes that Nature has developed to keep our species going for hundreds of thousands of years. We will be in charge of our own evolution. Can we improve in just a few short years what it took Nature millions of years to perfect?

Our greatest asset, our ability to learn, may turn out to be our greatest liability as well. Once humans discover a new field for learning, it is like dangling a carrot in front of the donkey. Humans as learning machines cannot resist the temptation to learn. As our desire for mental stimulation leads us into uncharted territory, we proceed because we crave knowledge of our world, and we need to know what happens around the next turn in the road. If we should have stopped now and not proceeded down that last stretch of road, we will probably never know except in hind sight. Then we can say, "Oh, yeah, we shouldn't have gone there," and try frantically to compensate for our error in judgment.

Fiddling with the genetic processes that took so long to create is indeed a mind boggling enterprise. It is a field that requires researchers with a strong sense of responsibility to humanity not researchers driven by the bottom line. No one would want to be the scientist who takes the plunge and makes the mistake that is fatal to humanity or wreaks havoc on the planet. Experimentation with life and genetics is a dangerous undertaking.

Genetic engineering takes genetic information encoded on our genes by means of DNA (deoxyribonucleic acid) and uses that material as a resource to be manipulated and changed. The three areas where genetic engineering is most useful are in basic research on gene structure and function, production of useful proteins by new methods, and generation of transgenic (genetically altered) plants and animals, says Desmond Nicholl in *Genetic Engineering*.

With genetic engineering, a new term *genethics* has been coined to deal with the ethical problems that arise. These problems, according to Nicholl, are going to increase in number and complexity as the genetic engineering program gets more advanced and has more applications. For instance, who owns seeds that have been genetically engineered? The public or a private company? A farmer cannot raise patented plants by seed unless they are purchased from the creating company. It remains to be seen if genetic engineering will be used for the overall benefit of mankind or some individual's economic profits.

For background information, some of the most important steps of genetics have occurred quite recently. In the early 1900s, Mendel experimented with peas and how they propagated. In 1953, the discovery of the structure of DNA by James Watson and Francis Crick was a milestone in work at the molecular level. In 1967, the enzyme DNA ligase was isolated which acts like glue to hold two strands of DNA together. This material is a necessary to glue to different pieces of DNA together to make a new genetic combination.

On the other hand, in 1970, a restriction enzyme was discovered which enables scientists to cut the DNA at precisely defined sequences. (An enzyme is defined as a catalyst that causes reactions of the chemicals of metabolism in living organisms.) With the discovery of the means to cut DNA and the means to glue different combinations together, the field of genetic engineering was ready to take off. Genes are composed of DNA. "It is a remarkable fact than an organism's characteristics are encoded by a four-letter alphabet, defining a language of three-letter words," says Nicholl. The basic four components of the 4-letter alphabet include the bases : adenine (A), guanine (G), cytosine (C) and thymine (T). Different combinations of these substances create the different genes that occur in living organisms.

A successful gene meets certain criteria. What does a gene need to be successful through time? (1) It needs to be stable enough to function in a living organism for up to 100 years or more. (2) The gene must be capable of making copies of itself to be passed on to future generations or it becomes a dead end. (3) The successful gene needs to have the potential for limited alteration of genetic material in order for the organism to change when necessary and to progress up the evolutionary ladder, says Nicholl.

Genes, the basic unit of genetic information, are then found on chromosomes. The DNA molecule of which genes are made, is a double helix. Each strand of the helix can store genetic data but in most organisms only one strand is used to encode any one gene.

For genetic engineering, the first necessity is to isolate the unit of genetic material that the person wants to put in another genetic spot. The source of this material is nucleic acid which is found either in DNA or RNA (Ribonucleic Acid). DNA and RNA materials can be found in any virus, bacteria, plant, or animal, but the cell has to be opened to get the nucleic acid out. "The method used to open cells should be as gentle as possible, preferably utilizing enzymatic degradation of cell wall material (if present) and detergent lysis of cell membranes," writes Nicholl. Basically, the scientist has to be as gentle as possible in getting the genetic material out of the cell without mangling it so badly that it cannot be used.

To greatly simplify matters, after various washing processes the DNA or RNA in the nucleic acid is put into an emulsion with ethanol and placed in a centrifuge. After spinning in the centrifuge, the various ingredients in the solution concentrate out at different levels. Then, the DNA or RNA can be collected from the different levels to start the process of genetic engineering.

Once the DNA is cut and pasted into another strand of genetic material it becomes usable to the new organism. In order to follow the new genetic material and see where it goes in the organism, it is tagged with a radioactive molecule. These radioactive molecules can then be traced to see the route the new genetic material has followed, what system it becomes incorporated into, and what has been the result.

Transgenic animals, that have been altered genetically, pose one of the most complex aspects of genetic engineering, both because of technical difficulty and because of the ethical problems that arise as a result. Many people who accept the genetic manipulation of bacteria, fungus, and plant species as beneficial, find difficulty in extending this acceptance when animals (particularly mammals) are involved. The need for sympathetic and objective discussion of this topic by the scientific community, the media and the general public is likely to present one of the great challenges in scientific ethics over the next few years, says Nicholl.

Some of the proposed benefits of transgenic animals would be to modify genes to cure cancer, a worthy goal. Farm animals could be genetically altered to achieve desirable traits, but the genetically altered traits would be desirable for humans not necessarily for the animal that is receiving the manipulated gene. For example, a growth hormone gene was introduced into a pig, and it showed greater food efficiency and lower concentrations of fat, but it also had an enlarged heart, stomach ulcers, dermatitis, kidney disease, and arthritis. Clearly, a few more bugs need to be ironed out before the process is going to work very well with animals or people.

Star-link corn, a genetically altered corn, is now being grown by farmers. It has been approved for use in pet food but not for human consumption. Yet, it is being used in products intended for humans without anyone knowing exactly what the effects will be. It has been noticed that monarch butterflies are killed by the pollen from these corn flowers. Keeping tabs on these products may be a tough job. It may be that these genetically altered products are better for the companies creating them than they are for the society as a whole or the receiver organism.

Furthermore, there is the problem that when the genetic code of humans becomes so well defined, will it remain private? Will clients be denied health insurance if the insurance company discovers that they have a gene for cancer or some other dangerous, expensive disease?

There is, of course, the possibility of cloning humans, both for reproduction and for spare body parts. So far, the technology for cloning is not reliable enough for human use. Some clones of animals have died early or not matured correctly. As cloning pioneers Rudolf Jaenisch and Ian Wilmut have argued, "if human cloning is attempted, those embryos that do not die early may live to become abnormal children and adults, both are troubling outcomes." quotes Sarah Richardson in "The Waiting List for Clones." Germany, France, Japan, and Australia currently have bans on human cloning, says Richardson.

According to Joseph Coates, these are some of the developments that we can look for in the next century: We will be able to grow neurons in a dish and alter them biochemically to make them do what we want.

Better and more thorough treatment of brain diseases due to the advances in brain research and technology will be available. Many disorders will be prevented or successfully treated such as aggression, addiction, learning problems, depression, schizophrenia, degenerative disease, dementia, and others associated with aging, stress, obesity, hypertension, and pain. Control of cognitive ability, mood, and memory may be possible.

Genetic engineering is a process that is here to stay. It will be refined and used, for better or for worse. Viruses, bacteria, plants, and animals (including humans) can all be genetically altered. The question is whether it will be beneficial or dangerous.

Man/Machine Combinations

Humans are going to have to conquer outer space at some point or the human race will go extinct as the sun burns out, explodes, and incinerates a good part of the solar system. Humans will have to modify themselves either genetically, with a process like freezing, or combine human and machine in order to make the extremely long voyages required to reach the closest destinations in outer space. This is with the present understanding that we won't be able to travel much faster than the speed of light, if that fast. If another speedier method of space travel is developed then the necessity to modify the human could change.

The age of science fiction is here. We are on the threshold of a new age. Many space ships in science fiction stories had a huge computer that was part machine and part human who was practically omniscient. High tech is becoming more efficient in combining the benefits of human and machine. Since the human is an elctro/chemical being; it is possible to combine it with an electric machine. We will probably live to see e-humans, humans that have been electronically enhanced.

If pollution in the environment becomes so hazardous that humans can't live; it might be that human/machine combinations will be the only survivors of a major pollution disaster. Or, if the climate changes so drastically that humans can't survive, the machine combinations might be a real possibility. However, no one expects any of these calamities to happen in the near future.

If computers take over so much of the human processes of memory, intelligence, and logic; it could be possible that the human brain will change drastically to accommodate these new situations. The uses of the brain might veer off in an entirely unanticipated direction.

The technology is within sight of humans being able to control machines, especially computers by thought and brain signals. Canadian Corporate News reports that IBVA or Interactive Brainwave Visual Analyzer which reads brain waves and amplifies them so that they may trigger movies, music, home automation devices, images, sounds, other software or almost any electronically addressable device. These abilities will be especially beneficial for the physically handicapped.

The capacity to build artificial neurons and electronic brains is not far off. But the question arises, how complex do we them to be? Do we want machines that might ultimately be smarter than humans? Humans are restricted by the size of the brain that must fit through the birth canal but an e-brain is not. An e-brain, an electronic brain, could reach unlimited size and complexity without the constraints put on humans by biology, says Paul Anthony in *Fortune Magazine*. Scientists need to be careful that they can control what they create.

Regular products will take on new and different roles. Refrigerators will tell us when to buy milk. A Smart Toilet produced by Matsushita Electric Industrial Company of Japan is designed to test a person's temperature, blood pressure, and blood sugar, reports Rob Kaiser in the *Chicago Tribune*. These innovations will completely change our way of life and the medical system. "In 5 to 10 years time, this could replace your doctor," says Michio Kaku, professor of theoretical physics at City University of New York.

There is currently the capacity to use computer chips, slightly larger than a quarter, embedded in the human to store ID and medical information in case of an emergency, writes David Streitfeld in the *Los Angeles Times*. The patient would be scanned like a can of tomatoes at the grocery store and the computer would retrieve vital information about his or her health, allergies, medicines and other crucial information in an emergency room situation. This technology would benefit Alzheimer patients who wander off and cannot be identified. It would help law enforcement in countries where there are a lot of kidnappings. Controversy may arise over who in the future might receive the chip. It could easily be misused.

Cyborg "Ratbots" which are special rats with electrodes embedded in their brains can be guided to search for buried victims in catastrophes like the September 11 bombings. This research alarms animal welfare people who claim that it is not good for the rats and that people are just regarding the rest of the animals on earth as potential tools for our control, writes Mark Henderson in the *Times*. We are on the edge of monumental changes in our society and way of life. Our ability to adapt, the ability of the brain to rise to different levels, will be a world wide challenge for the human race and ultimately the rest of life on the planet. The human brain in its search for learning, knowledge, and stimulation will find many opportunities and create many hazards.

It is interesting to speculate what role exactly that humans are destined to fill here on planet earth. Probably the most imaginative has the best chance of being right. Since viruses have been here since the beginning (about four billion years), and since humans are relative newcomers to the planet; we are probably the vehicle whereby the virus will travel to the next solar system before this solar system burns out. Eistein said something to the effect that independence is the conceit of consciousness. We think we are independent because we are conscious. Yet we are all connected; we just do not know what role we are playing.

Appendix 213

TOPICS TO CONSIDER

1. DO YOU FEEL THAT SCIENTISTS ARE ENTERING DANGEROUS TERRIROTY WITH GENETIC ENGINEERING?

2. SHOULD THE ADVANCEMENT OF MACHINES BE LIMITED IN SOME WAY?

3, WOULD YOU WANT TO CLONE YOURSELF?

4. IN THE NEW WORLD OF MAN/MACHINE COMBINATIONS, WITH WHAT MACHINE WOULD YOU LIKE TO INTERACT?

5. IF THE TECHNOLOGY WERE POSSIBLE, WHEN YOU DIE, WOULD YOU LIKE TO LIVE ON AS PART OF A MACHINE?

6. SHOULD HUMANS DO GENETIC MANIPULATION OF THEMSELVES?

7. IF YOU HAD THE CHOICE, WOULD YOU MAKE YOUR CHILDREN OUTSTANDING IN SOME SPECIFIC AREA? IS THIS ETHICAL?

Appendix II
BRAIN IMAGE TECHNOLOGY

It is only through new technology that modern advances in the study of the brain have become possible. PET (positron emission tomography) and MRI (Magnetic Resonance Imaging) are modern methods that enable scientists to see which areas of the brain are active during specific activities and behaviors. With these new methods, neuroscientists look at the brain as it works. Scientists are able to take photographs that show different brain areas lit up and are therefore able to see which areas of the subject's brain are active. New Methods permit the study of the living brain where the subject talks to the researchers or performs certain assigned tasks while being observed.

PET (positron emission tomography) and fMRI (functional magnetic resonance imaging) measure brain activity. PET shows that more active parts of the brain burn more glucose, a type of sugar that the brain uses for energy. In PET scans the brain is injected with radioactive glucose and the scan traces which parts of the brain are burning up this tagged glucose. The fMRI measures which areas of the brain are activited by looking at blood flow and the use of oxygen. The fMRI doesn't involve injections and can be used with children.

In a Public Broadcasting Series called *Secret Life of the Brain*, scientists describe how the MRI works. It takes a clear and detailed picture of the brain often in cross-sections that look like slices. The MRI sends a radio impulse through an area of the brain which makes certain atoms spin at a particular frequency (speed) and in a particular direction. The spin and frequency are different for every different type of tissue. When the radio pulse is turned off, the atoms return to their original position and release energy. It is this released energy that forms the signal that the MRI machine picks up. The signals are sent to a computer which processes the signals and creates a picture of the different types of tissue involved.

The magnetic field of the MRI runs straight down the machine and down the patient's body. This causes the hydrogen atoms in the head to all face in one direction, thus allowing for the slice view of the tissue.

MEG or magnetoencephalography detects the

faint magnetic fields that come from brain activity. The brain's magnetic field is translated in a very sensitive instrument called the SQUID or superconducting quantum interference device. Of all the scanning methods MEG gives the best resolution and accuracy. The only drawbacks are these huge machines weigh about 98 tons and cost in the multimillions.

These new technologies show the complex relationship between the different parts of the brain in action, and which parts of the brain work together for any one function. They show reactions of the brain over time as it is receiving stimuli through the senses. These technologies enable scientists to see the brain in action and have provided enormous leaps in the understanding of how the brain works.

However, the field of brain scanning is relatively new and some have reservations as to what exactly is being measured. Just because a certain area is lit up may not mean it is thinking. What if the lit up or active area were just carrying out the waste products left over from the area that is thinking. Some believe that it is uncertain as to what exactly is being measured in brain scans.

Notes

Lauretta DeForge, the author, is a student of literature and the arts. She has a BA degree in English with a minor in French and an MA in Linguistics. She has spent many happy hours studying foreign language, especially French.

The arts have always been a major part of her life, since early chilhood she has been liberally supplied with paper, pencils, and paint. Lauretta has done drawing, painting in oil, acrylics, and water colors. The author enjoys doing pottery, mosaics, and playing the piano. Matter of fact, she currently teaches piano. She loves music as a composer, piano player, choir participant, dancer, and listener. Her creativity has brought her enormous personal satisfaction and emotional reward.

Lauretta is an avid dancer. She did folk dancing for more than 20 years and considers that to be one of the best experiences of her life. The author now does contra dancing and ballroom dancing as a major hobby. The author tries to keep active, being a lover of exercise. She currently adds hiking and swimming to her love of dance. She loves hiking and cross-country skiing in the forests of the Northwest.

The author loves beauty, both as a creater and appreciator of it. She enjoys walking through beautiful gardens. For her, a house is not a home until the art work goes up inside and gardens are established outside. Beautiful and bright colors add spice to life and make her feel more cheerful.

The author also likes to write, hence the impetus for the book. She uses a journal just to keep in writing practice. Writing is the way to pass what she knows to the next generation and to share her love of art with others.

In the year 2000, the author became interested in the workings of the human brain. She attended many of the lectures presented by Oregon Health Sciences University at the Oregon Museum of Science and Industry. This field is changing dramatically even as the reader finishes this book. The human brain remains a fascinating study.

This book was born out of the desire to live life as fully as possible and to determine how best to accomplish that goal. This book advocates fulfillment by way of creativity and the arts, plus all the necessities of the happy, healthy brain. The author touches on what it takes to make a happy human: a goal that we all strive to reach.

BIBLIOGRAPHY

Ackerman, Diane. *A Natural History of the Senses.* Vintage Books, New York. 1990.

Allman, John. *Evolving Brains.* Scientific American Library, New York. 2000.

Anthony, Paul. "I Compute, Therefore I am," *Fortune* (Asia). Feb 7, 2000. Vol. 141 Issue 3, p20.

Appleton, Leroy. *American Indian Design and Decoration.* Dover Publiscation, New York. 1971.

Arnhein, Rudolph. *Visual Thinking.* University of California Press, Berkeley. 1997.

Bayles, David and Ted Orland. *Art and Fear.* The Image Continuum. Eugene, Or. 1993.

Begley, Sharon. "Religion and the Brain" in *Newsweek*, May 7, 2001.

Birks, Tony. *The Complete Potter's Companion.* Bulfinch Press, Boston. 1993.

Bisignani, J. *Hawaii Handbook.* Moon Publications, California. 1995.

Boysson-Bardies, Benedicte de. *How Language Comes to Children.* A Bradford Book, Cambridge. 1999.

Brown, Denise, *Massage.* Teach Yourself Books, Coventry, England. 1996.

Campbell, Don. *The Mozart Effect.* Willian Morrow. 1995.

Canadian Corporate News. **Stephen Hawkings Remarks Gives Giant Boost to Brain/Computer Interface Maker IBVA Technologies.** Sept 10, 2001.

Coates, Joseph. "Brain Technology on Way," *Research Technology Management,* May/June, 1995.

Cousins, Norman. *Anatomy of an Illness.* Bantam Books, New York. 1979.

Davis, Gary. *Creativity is Forever.* Kendall/Hunt Publishing Co., Iowa, 1986.

Damasio, Antonio and Hanna Damasio. "Brain and Language" *Scientific American.*

Dean, Ward. John Moargenthaler, Steven Fowkes, *Smart Drugs II.* Smart Publications, California. 1993.

DeBecker, Gavin. *The Gift of Fear.* Dell Books, New York. 1997.

Diamond, Jared. *Guns, Germs, and Steel.* Norton, New York. 1997.

Diamond, Jared. *The Third Chimpanzee.* Harper Perenniel, New York. 1992.

Domar, Alice. *Self-Nurture.* Penguin Books, New York. 2000.

Drubach, Daniel. *The Brain Explained.* Prentice Hall Health, New Jersey. 2000.

Edwards, Betty. *Drawing on the Right Side of the Brain.* Penguin, Putnam, New York. 1999.

Gardner, Howard. *The Arts and Human Development.* Basic Books, New York. 1994.

Gardner, Howard. *Multiple Intelligences.* Basic Books, New York. 1993.

Glancey, Jonathan. *The Story of Architecture.* DK Publishing, New York. 2000.

Glausiusz, Josie. *"The Mystery of Music," Discover.*

Goldsmith, Joan. *How Can We Keep From Singing.* Norton and Co., London. 2001.

Gopnik, Alison, Andrew Meltzoff, and Patricia Kuhl. *The Scientist in the Crib.* Morrow, New York. 1999.

Haseltine, Eric. *"Fear and Evolution,"* Discover. August, 2001.

Healy, Jane. *Endangered Minds*. Simon and Schuster, New York. 1990

Henderson, Mark. "Remote Control Rat will Beat Lassie to the Rescue," *The Times,* May 2, 2002.

Heyerdahl, Thor. *Kon Tiki*. Washington Square Press, New York. 1984.

James, John, and Frank Cherry. *The Grief Recovery Handbook*. Harper Perenniel, New York. 1988.

Kaiser, Rob. "Japanese Firm's Smart Toilet Is Just a Sign of Future Technology," *Chicago Tribune,* Dec 22, 2000.

Katsh, Shelley and Carol Merle-Fishman. *The Music Within You*. Simon and Schuster, New York. 1985.

Klawans, Harold. *Defending the Cavewoman.* Norton and Co., New York. 2000.

Kotulak, Ronald. *Inside the Brain.* Andrews McMeel, Kansas City. 1997.

Kramlinger, Keith. *Mayo Clinic on Depression.* Mayo Foundation, New York. 2001.

Lewis, Thomas, Fari Amini, Richard Lannon. *A General Theory of Love.* Vintage Books, New York. 2001.

Maess, Burkhard. Science, "Music, Language, May Meet in the Brain." as reported in *Science News*, May 5, 2001.

Malchiodi, Cathy. *The Art Therapy Source Book.* Lowell House, Los Angeles. 1998.

Morgan, Elaine. *The Aquatic Ape.* Stein and Day, New York. 1982

Nicholl, Desmond. *Genetic Engineering.* Cambridge University Press, England. 1994.

Niele, Caren. "Storytelling," *The Toastmaster.* July, 2001.

Ornstein, Robert. *Evolution of Consciousness.* Touchstone Book, New York. 1991.

Pickering, Jerry. *Theatre.* West Publishing Company, St. Paul. 1978.

Prend, Ashley. *Transcending Loss.* Berkley Books, New York. 1997.

Provine, Robert. *Laughter.* Viking, New York. 2000.

Ratey, John. *A User's Guide to the Brain.* Pantheon Books, New York. 2001.

Restak, Richard. *Modular Brain.* MacMillan Publishing Co., New York, 1994.

Restak, Richard. *Mozart's Brain and the Fighter Pilot.* Three Rivers Press, New York. 2001.

Restak, Richard. *The New Brain.* Rodale Press, New York. 2003.

Richman, Linda. *I'd Rather Laugh.* Warner Books, New York. 2001

Richardson, Sarah. "The Waiting List for Clones, " *Discover,* Jan 2002, Vol 23, Issue 1, p68.

Ridley, Matt. *The Red Queen.* Penguin Books, New York. 1993.

Scott, Alwyn. *Stairway to the Mind.* Springer-Verlag, New York, 1995.

Secunda, Victoria. *Losing Your Parents, Finding Yourself.* Hyperion, New York. 2000.

Streitfeld, David. "First Humans to Receive ID Chips," *Los Angeles Times,* May 9, 2002.

Thayer, Robert. *The Origin of Everyday Moods.* Oxford University Press. New York, 1996.

Tomatis, Alfred. *The Conscious Ear.* Station Hill Press, N.Y. 1991.

Washnis, George and Richard Hricak. *Discover of Magnetic Health.* Nova Publish Co, Maryland, 1993.

Walsh, David. *Selling Out America's Children.* Fairview Press, Minneapolis. 1995.

Walsh, David. *Cyberhood.* Simon and Schuster, New York. 2001.

Wright, Karen and Ralph Steadman. *"The Sniff of Legend," Discover,* April, 1994.

Zeki, Semir. "The Visual Image in Mind and Brain," *Scientific American.* American Lyons Press, New York. 1999.

Index

A
Acting 116
Aggression 123
Aquatic ape 13,15
Architecture 149
Art definition 105
Art therapy 108

B
Babies 61
Boring work 52
Brain activities 174
Brain Changes 14, 20
Brain Evolution 6
Brain scan 214
Building Arts 149

C
Children and Art 84
Chimpanzee 7
Choral music 137
Coping skills 199
Couple dancing 156
Creativity 89

D
Dance 156
Death 46
Depression 51
Diet p. 177
Divorce 44
Drama 116
Drawing 139

E
Emotional system 9-10
Euphoria of creation 94
Eye 23

F,
Fixation 37

G
Genetically altered humans 201
Genetic engineering 201

H
Hearing 30

I
Incubation 91
Illumination 91

J,K,L
Language 72, 79, 194
Left brain 92
Laughter 190
Learning 61
Limbic system 9
Love 36

M
Man/machine combination 209
Memory 55
Mood 39
Movement 155
Mozart effect 130
Music 129

N
Neotony 17
Neuron 7-8
New born 61
New brain 71

O, P
Order blank 232
Painting 139
Perspective 140
Physical movement 155
Piano 135
Positive thinking 176
Pottery 151
Preparation 91
Public speaking 115

Q, R
Reading 116
Reptile brain 9

S
Savannah 13
Sculpture 151
Seeker 100
Senses 19
Sensory Deprivation 111, 44, 53, 183
Sex 119
Sight 23
Singing 136
Sleep 58
Social contact 187
Spirituality 162
Sports 159
Storytelling 113

T
Tickling 29
Touch 27
TV 67

U,V
Verification 91
Veteran 102
Visual artist 145
Vitamins 180

WXYZ
Writing 117

ORDER FORM

Fax Orders 503-646-9573

Phone Orders 503-646-9573

Postal Orders

DeForge Communications
http://home.
netcom.com
/ldeforge/

Please send the following book: *Art Smart*

Name ―――――――――――――――

Address ――――――――――――――

City ―――――――――――――――――

State ―――――― Zip ――――――

Telephone ―――――――――――――

Email Address ―――――――――
Please add sales tax if applicable.

	No. of books	Total price
Art Smart ($12.00 each)		
Standard shipping per book		3.50
Final Total		